That's Unacceptable!

Surviving a Brain Tumor
My Personal Story

By
Rebecca L. Libutti

Krystal Publishing
1997

Krystal Publishing, September, 1997

NOTE TO THE READER: The information contained in this book is based upon personal experience. It is not intended nor should it be construed as a substitute for consulting with your physician. All matters regarding your health require medical supervision.

Cover and printing: Jeff Stein, Incentives USA, Inc.
Scotch Plains, New Jersey

The author is grateful for permission to reprint the following copyrighted materials:

Rebecca Libutti: Recovery Unlimited printed in Search newsletter of the National Brain Tumor Foundation in San Francisco, CA

Photograph on page 190 is courtesy of Gene Gabelli Studios in Verona, New Jersey.

Printed in the U.S.A.

Dedication

Dedicated to my daughter, Krystal Lee Libutti, whose big brown eyes and contagious smile are filled with compassion and understanding, whose warm heart and warm hands have filled my life with purpose, and whose uncanny humor has filled my heart with laughter. You have given me the courage to go on and on and on... my true energizer.

And to Warren ... what can I say? You are the answer to my prayers and the light at the end of the long dark tunnel. You have given me strength and courage and determination along with an endless love that will endure for eternity.

Many thanks, with my warmest appreciation and love to my family whose loving support is my greatest comfort; thank you Mom and Dad, Lillian, Michele, Renzo, Mick, Cindy, Brian, Lori, Jodi, John, Marissa, Marc, Paul, Katie, Justin, Benjamin, Mackenzie, and Cameron.

And a special hug and thanks to Mackenzie who at two years old, has endured more than any child or adult I have ever known and yet she smiles, she laughs, she giggles as she waits patiently for a better life. May we all learn from her that "there remain faith, hope, love, these three; but the greatest of these is love." First Corinthians 13:13(NWT)

Thank you to each and every friend, silver and golden, old and new, here and there, who have made the journey worth the struggle.

My apologies to all others for sounding like I'm accepting the Oscar at the Academy Awards.

Acknowledgment

There are far more people to thank and far too few pages to acknowledge all. Among the many, I wish to thank Virginia Shrodo for her endless encouragement to complete this book and for her support in making it a reality. Her editing was invaluable to this endeavor. I also wish to thank Dr. Brian Beyerl, for without his skill and compassion, this book might be missing its present author. Dr. Beyerl, in my book you have achieved a summit far greater than the highest mountain and for that I will be eternally grateful. To Patricia Phillips, R.N., for the courage and inspiration her support group provides to all of us coping with a brain tumor. To Ann Short Chirhart for her editing and critiquing and her positive words encouraging me to continue. To Jeff Stein who lended his expertise, his resources, and a listening ear to get this book to publication. To Eileen Mullen, aka Nurse, for extending a helping hand and resources to acheive our goal. To Betsy Gravett whose generosity made the load lighter for us all. And, to Dr. Mark Malkin for giving me hope when the horizon was so far away.

Foreword

When our son was diagnosed with a malignant brain tumor in 1991, we scoured our local library for any books on the subject. Except for a few excerpts in medical texts we found nothing more recent than John Gunther's *Death Be Not Proud*, and I had read that as a teenager. It was frustrating not to have access to a book that would provide us with both information and hope. We would have jumped for joy had we been able to find anything like Rebecca Libutti's *That's Unacceptable*.

This book is a gift. Rebecca has filled it with the story of her battle against a glioblastoma multiforme. She has included what it feels like to be told you have a terminal disease; she has taken us through the periods of ups and downs, of laughter and tears; she has stuffed the pages with the realities of waging war against this foreign invader while dealing with the feelings and fears of family and friends. She has given practical opinions on how to deal with the doctors, nurses, hospitals, alternative practitioners and insurance companies. She has included passages filled with faith and humor as well as stark realities. And she has taken this book-- this gift-- and wrapped it in hope.

This is a book that some of us have waited a life time for and is equally precious to brain tumor survivors, their caregivers, their loved ones, their medical teams as well as anyone who is facing a life altering situation. So read this book, and accept the gift that Rebecca has given to you. You cannot remain unchanged in your feelings and attitude after finishing it. By sharing in her journey, you, too, become a survivor. Anything else is unacceptable

- Virginia Shrodo

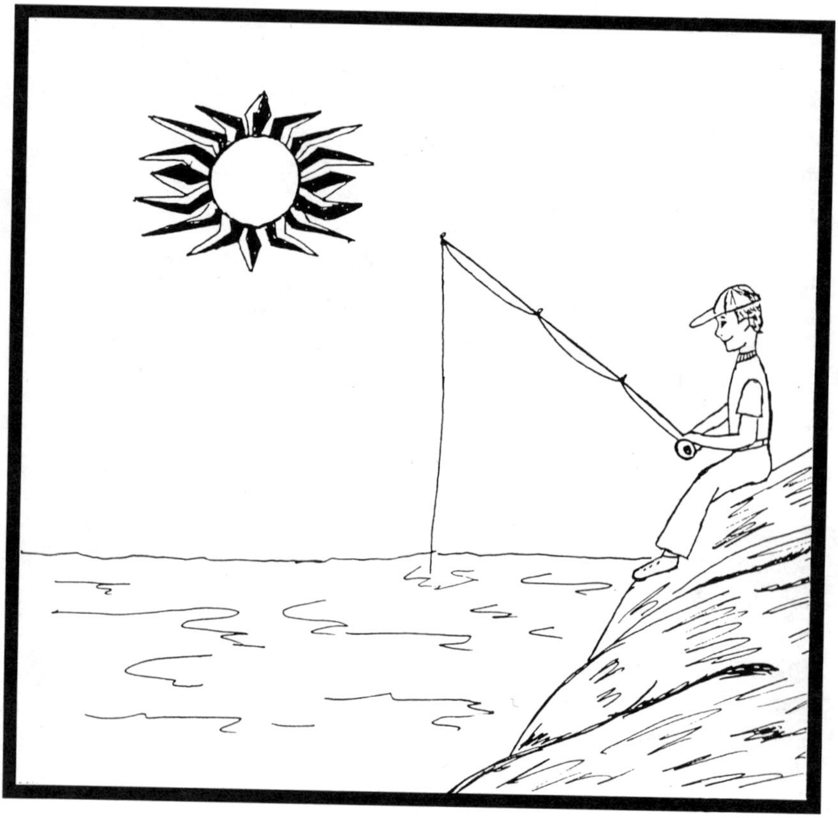

Gone Fishin'

In Heart and Memory

This book was written with the ever-present thoughts of the friends I met along the way, friends I knew only too briefly, and some I hope to meet in a kinder world. It is written in memory of:

Matt, who's gone fishin';

Frank, who's rollerblading without a helmet;

Brian, who's running in the sunshine;

Linda, who's walking with the clouds;

Marj, whose soprano permeates the universe with joy; and

Maureen, whose beauty and warmth remains in our hearts.

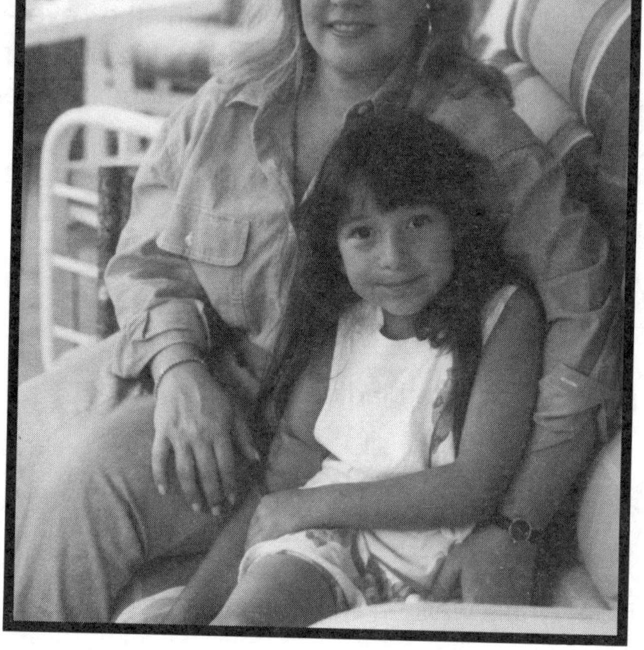

July, 1993 - Life Before The Brain Tumor
Rebecca and Krystal Libutti

Introduction

Allow me to invite you into my world. It is a mystery to most of my friends and acquaintances; for others it is all too real. I want you to close your eyes and imagine your wife, your sister, your daughter - 38 years young, strong and healthy - when suddenly a doctor says "she has a brain tumor."

Now you are standing in my shoes. What do YOU do? How do YOU feel?

Not only do you have a brain tumor, but it is malignant - not encapsulated. It is the most aggressive of all cancers and you are literally 'losing your mind.' They tell you there is no known cause, no known cure, and treatments are ineffective at best.

Now you are walking in my shoes. Where do YOU find strength, what coping skills do YOU use? How does it feel?

You are told the odds are you will live less than one year. You are rushed into an emergency craniotomy, with layer after layer of your skull peeled open, to reach deep into the cavern of your brain and remove a cancer whose cells double themselves every 21 days.

Your worst nightmare plays out in real life. Where do you turn for comfort, for solace, for support?

You must endure daily radiation treatments for seven weeks, followed by harsh chemotherapy treatments for 11 months.

Now you have walked a mile in my shoes. Is YOUR faith strong enough to carry you? Is YOUR conviction powerful enough to lift you up against the odds? Can you ever feel safe when your own body has betrayed you - can you trust it will not fail again?

Each night you lay your head on your pillow and it is with you. Can you sleep in peace? Every morning it is there to greet you. Can you ignore it? You must conquer it, for to accept it is unacceptable.

Enter my world, not to be frightened, but to become strong for me; not to become depressed, but to be hopeful to help me stay positive; not to be downhearted but to be uplifted by an indomitable spirit we can share; not to walk in my shoes, but to walk beside me and share my journey.

Table of Contents

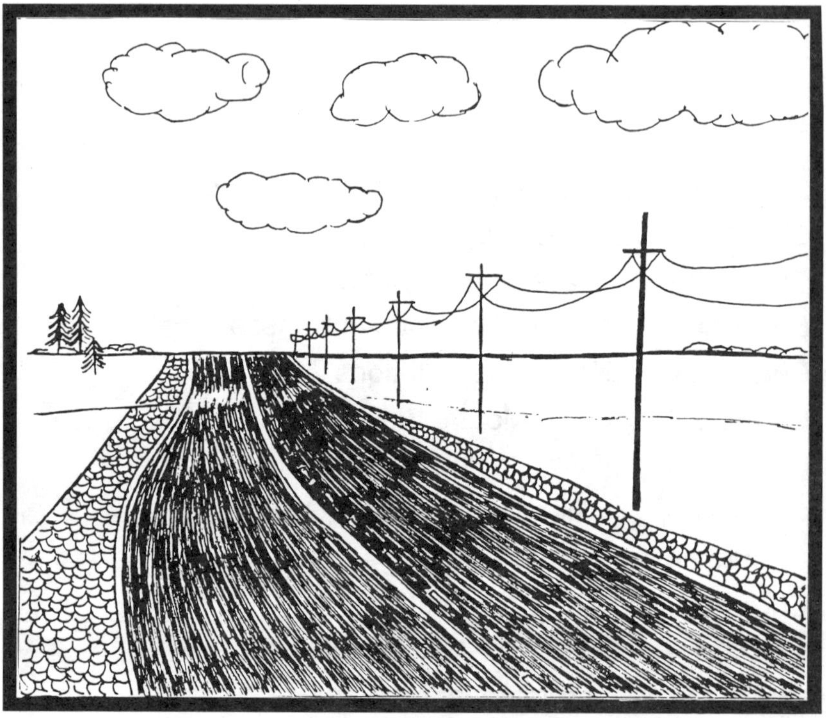

The Journey Begins

A Journey of a Thousand Miles Begins

I should have suspected something was wrong that Friday, September 17, 1993 when I arrived at my new office feeling a bit strange. I poured my usual cup of coffee and knew something was wrong when I put the coffee pot in the refrigerator and the milk on the burner. How wrong, was the farthest thing from my mind. After working for half a day, I figured I was getting the same flu that my daughter and husband had recently experienced, so I took the rest of the day off to try to get rid of this little "bug" before it got the better of me.

I laid low all weekend and was feeling fine and ready to return to work on Monday morning until at exactly 3:13 a.m., I awoke with the most excruciating headache of my life. The pain was in the front part of my head right where my sinus pain usually occurs. September is a particularly bad month for my allergies but even I knew this was no sinus headache. I could not lift my head off the pillow at 9:00 a.m. when I called my doctor's office. I begged them to have the doctor call me to prescribe something for the pain. I called three (3) times and literally cried on the phone that the pain was so intense I could not get to their office. They refused and said I must see the doctor. Since my husband had left for work, my neighbor John gave me a ride to my doctor's pristine Victorian home converted into a prestigious office for three physicians. I threw up on the front lawn - the pain now so severe.

I was examined and given medication for a sinus infection. Of course, my family physician knew I had just been there in May for a complete physical and $750.00 worth of blood work, all indicating I was in completely good health. So for three days I took the pills while the pain got worse. The intensity of the headache was located in the front of my head and it pierced straight through to my brain. It was excruciating to move an eyelid. For three days I kept the shades down, no radio, no TV, not even a whisper.

My sweet but usually overpowering Labrador Retriever, Murphy Brown, knew I was in pain and never once barked to go out. I am fanatical about my animals and I love them beyond belief, but I have one rule that had never before been broken - the animals are not allowed to get on my bed. Murphy is the most protective and watchful dog, though the biggest threat she poses to anyone is licking them to death. Since I took care of her and walked with her every day from the time she was a puppy, she had become my formal protector and guardian. By the third day, her senses told her that I was in great need of relief. With one determined bound, she jumped up onto my four-poster bed which requires a step stool for me to get on it. There she curled her warm body, gentle as a mother with a baby, right next to me, refusing to move the entire day. I will never forget the comfort this big gentle creature gave me when all those pills the doctor gave me could not.

The following day required another plea over the telephone, and once again I was flatly told it was imperative to make another visit to the office. Another neighbor, Linda, drove me to my doctor's office and this time she prescribed an extremely strong pain killer and set up a CT or CAT scan (Computerized Axial Tomography) indicating I might have a secondary infection.

The next day my husband, Warren, accompanied me for the scan. Since I was now feeling no pain, it was an easy task which I figured would detect my life long sinus and allergy problems were "all in my head". When the technician said my physician wanted me to take the scans to her office to review, I remember thinking, 'how odd' but since her office was only a few blocks away I didn't give it much more consideration. I was feeling no pain and expected her to tell me that "it" was over.

Instead, she looked quite distressed and uncomfortable. There was shaking in her voice when she asked me if the technicians had told me anything and she seemed to wince when I said, "No". Then she just blurted it out, "Rebecca, you have a mass on your brain and we do not know what it is." At first I laughed, thinking it was a warped medical joke but she wasn't laughing. Warren and I looked at each other in total confusion and both said in unison, "You must have gotten the wrong scans."

She simply said, "I have reserved a room for you at Overlook Hospital (as if I was going to a hotel). You need to go home and get packed and be there in an hour. There will be a neuro-surgeon waiting for you."

Within that 30 second statement, my life changed irrevocably. It was probably the first and last time throughout my ordeal that, just as promised, there was a surgeon waiting FOR ME! He was tall, dark, and handsome but the dream was all wrong! I remember thinking oddly, this kind of handsome rides in on a white horse not in a white medical coat; he plays strange music doing operations on episodes of ER; he rescues maidens in distress but I had already found my prince charming so what was HE doing here? This was soon to become my worst nightmare as the handsome neuro-surgeon in real life told me the real life news: I had a brain tumor ... a What?! That's a pretty hefty penalty for putting the coffee and milk in the wrong place, don't you think?

I never even heard of such a thing (not anyone I knew at least) and after almost twenty years underwriting life insurance, I thought I'd heard of nearly everything. What did I miss? Were there signs, symptoms, something, anything that might have foretold this kind of bizarre thing could happen to a happy, healthy, thirty-eight year-old mother and wife living peacefully (as peaceful as possible) in suburbia New Jersey?

Just the previous week I worked full-time preparing a twenty million dollar proposal, played three sets of tennis after work, baked cookies for my daughter's new second grade class, cooked, cleaned and cared for my family, went to my religious services and faithfully walked the dog. What happened to take me and my beloved family on this sharp turn of fate, fact or fiction?

Those questions were to be pondered in the days to come but for now there were other matters that required my attention. The neuro-surgeon explained that there was a mass (meaning tumor) on my brain. It could be a primary tumor which originated in the brain or a metastatic tumor which transferred from another part of the body. "It may or may not be operable", he said seriously. Whoa, slow down there, what language are you speaking?! I never heard any of these terms before and he might as well have been speaking Chinese for all I could understand. I felt fine, what was the big fuss? The whole world turned into one great cataclysmic blur. Maybe this was just a bad dream. Well, it was a bad dream and the worst part was, I was living it.

Throughout the following week, I underwent every kind of evaluation of every square and not so square inch of my anatomy to rule out the "M" thing which I was still unable to pronounce - metastasis or metastatic, meaning it originated elsewhere in the body and then moved to the brain. During this intense and disturbing battery of tests, my room filled with friends and family. The telephone rang incessantly with incoming calls from all over the country and as far away as Paris. A nurse came in to ask who was in the room because I was getting so many calls and visitors they were beside themselves. But the festivities in my room gave them a break and they stayed and ate and joined in the revelry with the rest of us.

By this point in time, however, I was paralyzed on the right side and could no longer sign consent for surgery. In place of my name, it was necessary to clutch the pen in my left hand and make a big "X". However, no one was certain surgery was an option. Tomorrow I would meet the neuro-surgeon and shake the hand (my left still worked) of the man who would help save my life.

Tomorrow came and with my husband, my father and mother at my side, in walked Dr. Brian Beyerl, a neuro-surgeon with specialized experience in stereotactic computer-assisted brain surgery. We listened as he described the needed craniotomy, more big words, blah, blah, more diffused words, blah, blah, blah. I understood the words brain surgery and tomorrow. I did not understand it was located deep in the left parietal lobe (sounds like an ear not a brain), I did not understand I could succumb to the surgery, it might not be successful, I might have a different personality (some I knew might vote for that), paralysis could remain, improve, or worsen and on and on the list of possibilities continued. I heard every word but nothing registered.

Suddenly everyone was gone from my room - probably some family conference in an effort to protect me. I looked up and there was Dr. Beyerl finishing up his notes on my hospital room door. I said, "What is your first name?" Without looking up, he said in a low monotone voice, "Bud". "Cute", I countered, "but you are not going to touch my brain until we are on a first name basis." He grinned, and as he left my room he said, "Brian, ... see you tomorrow."

Dr. Brian Beyerl was younger than I expected. When the doctor about to enter your brain is nearly the same age as you, it tends to rattle an already frazzled nerve.

Dr. Beyerl was extremely intelligent with a serious demeanor. Behind the wire rim glasses there was impressive intelligence which complemented his highly technical surgical skills. However, it was his hidden sense of humor that sold me. I found his serious side comforting because he was serious about helping me but the hint of humor let me know he was human and compassionate. He displayed a humble confidence and when he said, "I know I can do this", I replied with confidence, "Then let's do it!"

That evening I spent hours in the bathroom, talking to my image in the mirror and talking with God about my life. I desperately wanted to find a scripture from the Bible that I learned as a little girl. A very dear old friend called me an hour later. He was my minister from my home town and the man who showed me the scripture over twenty years ago. When I asked him if he remembered, although in his late seventies, he instantly recalled and said, "Isaiah Chapter 41 and verse 13" which says, "Do not be afraid, for I, Jehovah, your God, am grasping your right hand. I myself will help you." The very thought that God would even consider holding my hand brought me great comfort. I no longer felt I would be going into surgery alone - and who better to be with me?!

My spiritual mentor had always shared scriptures with me from as far back as I could remember and I had grown to love the Holy Bible with its wisdom and knowledge about my Creator. My friend now summed up my life-long studies, saying, "My dear, all your life you have known the scriptures, now you will come to understand them." It was a powerful statement and humbling to say the least. I knew that I was going to need the faith I had in my Creator to deal with the fight ahead. I prayed for hours until at last I felt an incredible peace come over me. It was no bright light, no rushing wind, no powerful voice from a crackling sky. It was serene and calm and internal. It was an absence of fear, replaced by a confidence in placing myself in God's hands and implicitly trusting His wisdom for the outcome. It is my belief that God does not will bad things upon us. I had nothing to do with this random act caused by human imperfection, therefore there was no guilt to contend with. It was believing with all my heart that I was not at fault or being tested for some ultimate purpose, nor did I think I was being called away from everything I loved as if I was needed more urgently somewhere else. I also believe that my intelligent Creator gave me a brain with the intention that I use it and now was a good time to start. I know that my belief system is not the same as another's. It is, however, where I found a great deal of comfort and strength and a powerful will to survive.

Warren sat next to me throughout the night in an uncomfortable arm chair, watching over me and no doubt fearful of what the coming morning might bring. My sleep, however, was divinely peaceful.

Morning arrived quietly. The bed rolled gently. I was escorted by the two most truly handsome men in my life, my husband, Warren, on one side and my Dad on the other. I was at peace. I said a silent prayer for God to guide the hands of my surgeon, to strengthen my loved ones, and to let me see my beautiful daughter again. It never occurred to me that it might have been otherwise.

Little did I know that I would have conversations throughout my surgery with the anesthesiologist (I guess they can't shut me up anywhere!). After surgery the anesthesiologist met my Dad and Warren in the halls and told them I did fine and he enjoyed working with me throughout surgery because I had a great sense of humor. I wish I could have taped THAT conversation!

Five hours later I was awakened by the soothing voice of the gentle nurses in the recovery room and then later the Intensive Care Unit. My surgeon came to see how much feeling I had and was pleased when I could move both feet and both arms and the only memory loss to date was the conversation with the anesthesiologist!

Soon they allowed Warren to see me and his face was beaming - I don't ever remember seeing him look so happy and relieved. My Dad followed, his exhaustion and relief combined in his warm smile and hug. Both were so proud of me and thrilled that I had come through this great ordeal so well. Mom and the rest of my sisters and brothers came in next and soon after the short visit, I fell back into a pleasant soothing sleep.

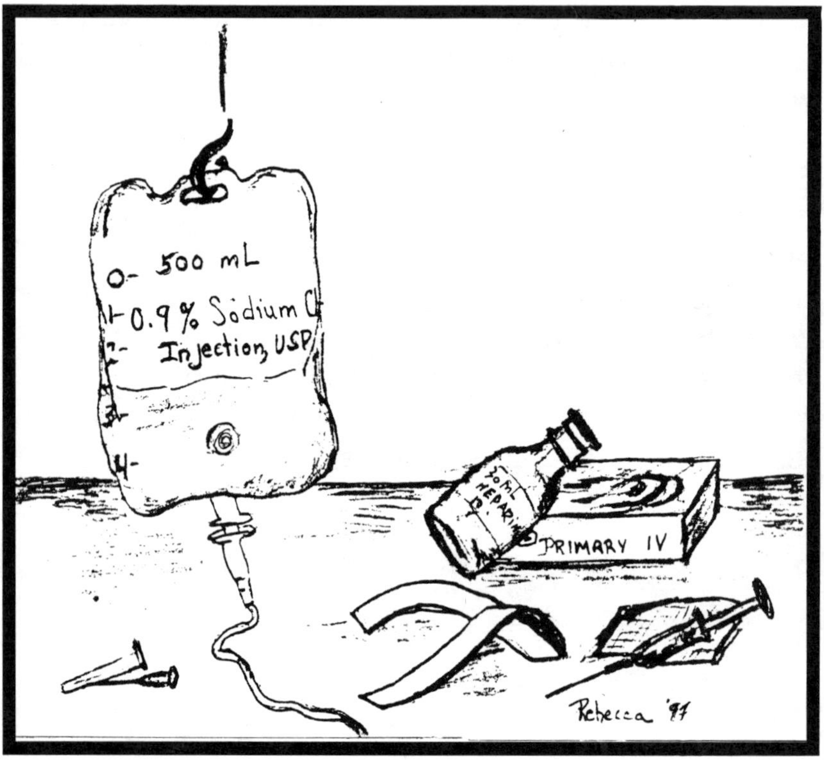

Reality Check

Mugged by Reality

After staying in ICU (the Intensive Care Unit) for less than twenty-four hours, the "real fun" began. I was "mugged by reality" when they moved me into a bright noisy room across from the nurses' station. My ninety year old room-mate was moaning and calling for a nurse as she needed a bed pan which did not arrive in time. This was the night-shift and it was scary.

I asked for a pain killer since the anesthesia was wearing off. The night nurse, unbeknownst to me, gave me Tylenol with Codeine even though I had specified I was allergic to codeine. After only a few hours post surgery, these delightful creatures had me violently vomiting next to the lady who wet the floor. They were so sympathetic, they left me lying in the vomit for some time along with the poor lady next to me in her wet bed. Somehow I kept wondering if the "call button" was set just out of my reach on purpose or was merely an oversight.

By morning I was in excruciating pain. My body ached from head to toe, the screw marks on my head from the iron "halo" began to throb. The iron halo is a device used during brain surgery to keep your head perfectly still while delicate surgery is being performed. My "halo" was attached to my head with screws which left a mark on my forehead for a few weeks but nothing too traumatic. It is intimidating looking but I prefer it to someone being responsible for holding me still while the surgeon operates for five or six hours.

Earlier that morning, in those wee morning hours when you don't function on a good day, nurses began taking vitals, checking tubes, drawing more blood.

With morning rounds beginning and the buzzing of the hospital as it begins a new day on the ninth floor NeuroScience Center, in strolls the covering physician. After finding that he prescribed the codeine because he didn't check my chart and was unavailable all night due to surgery, he no longer appeared so charming.

I begged for pain killers, Demerol and Percacet. An injection of Demerol, one quickly discovers, relieves pain instantaneously, and this "feel good, who cares what you look like" cocktail was beginning to feel wonderful. Never having smoked cigarettes or weed, never even remotely experimenting with non-prescription drugs, the strongest medications I tolerated were pediatric at best. But, ah, Demerol, I didn't even care that it required a needle to inject it. Give me more Demerol.

When the doctors and nurses began to feel I was just a little too in love with it, they switched me quickly to Percacet which also works wonders but at a much slower pace. One of the nurses suggested a morphine pump where you have a constant but controlled supply of pain killer to dose yourself. It is designed, however, to be self-regulated so you cannot overdose. My doctor advised against it, I guess not knowing whether he could trust me with such a device.

When I finally got the needed pain killers, I lay motionless for hours, feeling that all my energy and will had been sucked right out of me. I could hear movement around me but couldn't open my eyes. The next day I finally opened my eyes only to see the most somber anguished faces of all my immediate family staring at me, looking as if they were at a funeral. Each had their own prescription for my recovery and all with the best of intentions and none agreed on anything except their desire to see me well. I felt I was watching a colorized episode of the Twilight Zone, so I closed my eyes again and returned to la-la land.

Another day, I lay motionless. I felt beat up, closer to being run over by a Mack truck. I had no hunger, no thirst, only an ache in my throat which I later realized was from the tube they put down my throat during surgery. There seemed to be a growing concern around me but no one apparently knew what to do.

At some unlawful hour I was awakened to have four vials of blood drawn. A short time later another nurse came in for more blood for different tests. This time I protested in tears and this sweet pretty nurse tried valiantly to accommodate my request but was required to draw the blood anyway. As she began, suddenly she gasped, "Oh, are you Krystal's Mom?" I was jolted into reality. She continued softly, "I see her picture there and I know she is in the same class as my son, Ronnie." I was mortified by my appearance and instantly awakened to think of my little girl. I could not bear the thought of this woman I knew from school seeing me like this, never mind think of my daughter. The thought added to my agony.

When I woke later that morning, it was with a sense that I was not alone. At the foot of my bed stood my Dad quietly watching over me. He got up real early and brought coffee and just watched over me until I awoke. It was so comforting to see him there although it seemed like I was dreaming. He smiled to see me open my eyes and ask weakly for a sip of water. He held my hand and I felt so safe.

I am sure I could never know how difficult this was for him and my mother. I thought in that moment that there could only be one thing worse than my going through this ordeal, and that would be to have to watch my daughter endure it. My love for my Mom and Dad has always been strong as theirs has been for me, but in that momentary thought, I grew to love them even more. They drew up all their strength for me and for my husband and daughter, and in my father's eyes, I saw a lifetime of unconditional love.

I was even more grateful for his presence as it was time for another visit from the surgeon, but Dr. Beyerl was in surgery so I met with his partner who was increasingly concerned that I might (just maybe) be slipping into deep depression. Interesting concept, doc. After a medical pep-talk, he instructed the day nurse to assist him with removing the staples (did he say "staples?") and get me up and walking. After literally ripping the staples (in the same manner as one removes a band-aid) right out of my head and with all the gentleness of Attila the Hun, he left me with Marie, a strong but caring nurse whose experience in the day-to-day reality of the 9th floor, would be a welcomed relief for the duration of my stay.

Marie wheeled in a portable deluxe chair with an attached potty and told me to test drive it. I was recently informed by my dear Marie, that I was not the most cooperative patient at that moment in time. I can't imagine why but maybe, just maybe, I was indeed feeling sorry for myself. I was wondering silently, where was that nice guy with the wire rim glasses - Dr. Beyerl - who did the surgery? Why was I being lectured by his insensitive partner?

However, the pep talk served a purpose. It made me mad. Real mad. The kind of mad where I say, "I'll show you!" I got out of bed, and said to myself, "You wanna see walking, I'll show you walking!" I pulled away the privacy curtain and immediately flew down the hall, hospital gown flying in the wind revealing my back-end in motion for all to see.

With an orderly running after me trying to cover my derrière, my father doubled over with laughter at the spectacle, and me determined never to let go of my new found control - it was quite an exhibition. I guess I showed them - more than I intended - but effective nevertheless.

That was a turning point on the road to recovery. Come what may, this was my life, and I would never abdicate control to anyone. I was on my way to recovery and to becoming the biggest pain they had encountered in some time. I am convinced they enjoyed almost every minute of my stay and we all had some great moments during my visit at their 'resort hotel' on the hill.

Overlook Hospital is aptly named as it sits high on the top of the bordering Watchung Mountain Reservation in Summit, New Jersey. The 9th floor where neurosurgery patients dwell is quite nice and recently redone with rooms 'overlooking' the view of this prestigious town. There is an upscale community surrounding Overlook, and many lovely homes, buildings and high class shops.

I insisted on being moved to a room away from the nurses' station and got a double bonus: a room with a view and re-connected with my former roommate, Debbie, who had partied with us prior to my surgery. Debbie and I shared more than a room - we shared the trauma each was encountering as we awaited our respective surgeries and recoveries. It eased the pain for each of us - especially in those lonely dark hours at night. Although we have not seen each other since our hospital encounter, I will never forget the friendship we shared at that moment of crisis.

All that hallway activity, however, left me longing for my first shower. It was royal. I was able to discard that chintzy hospital gown for a cozy flannel (aren't hospital rooms cold? - well I was) pack my soap, powder, etc. and have a seat on the Shower Express to be escorted by Nurse Marie to the showers. She instructed me to stay seated and do NOT wet my head. She stood guard for a few minutes but soon left me in peace with all that water: warm, wonderful water. I never thought that clean water could do so much to refresh the soul, to heal a beaten spirit, and lift my heart. It was simply euphoric.

Nurse Marie returned three times before I would agree to leave this new found haven of tranquility. This became my daily ritual until Dr. Beyerl told me I had to go home because I was running up the hospital water bills. I knew I liked his sense of humor.

Nurse Marie had a gentler, kinder side and in a few days we became quite social. She was tough but more like a mother hen than a grizzly bear, as I initially perceived. All the nurses on the 9th floor were compassionate, kind, sensitive and caring. Many went out of their way for me and my family and I truly was grateful for the considerate care and professional support I received. I recently returned to see how they all were and let them know that their efforts were not in vain. My room had been converted into a conference room which I found quite fitting after all the medical conferences we held there.

I found Marie working that day. Some of the other nurses I remember had moved on, some were on leave, but my dear Marie remembered me and we reminisced about the showers. Dr. Beyerl walked in on the reunion and we chatted briefly. Everyone remembered the five pound box of Swiss chocolates I sent after my stay - even three years later nurses I did not recall personally fondly remembered those chocolates!

There is one more hospital event that turned the tide before I was to go home. It occurred shortly after surgery...

The Real Victor

"It is not the critic who counts, nor the man who points out how the strong man stumbles or where the doer of deeds could have done better. The credit belongs to the man who is actually in the arena, whose face is marred by the dust and sweat and blood, who strives valiantly, who errs and comes short again and again, and who at worst, if he fails, at least fails while daring greatly so that his place shall never be with those cold and timid souls who know neither defeat nor victory."

Theodore Roosevelt

THAT'S UNACCEPTABLE

Mom and I were walking the halls on this lovely warm September afternoon. The sun was shining so brightly and from the guest waiting room there was a panoramic view of the lovely Watchung Mountains. Being from New Hampshire originally, I never could really accept them as mountains but, nevertheless, a high point for New Jersey. My family from New England never saw so many deer and wild animals as they did on their daily drive through the reservation on route to the hospital.

Everyone was so proud of my walking and Mom and I would walk for short periods several times a day to keep me moving. This afternoon I was unexpectedly paged to return to my room. There was a radiologist in my room when we arrived. He introduced himself but I had some trouble understanding why he was there. It soon became clear.

The radiologist told me that I must begin radiation treatment immediately and he wanted to arrange for a date to begin. When I balked at the idea of taking immediate action, he tried to convince me by saying, "If you don't take the treatment, you will die in a year, and if you do, you will maybe live two years."

With Mom trying to hold me down, I started to rant and rave at him and the following words came out of my mouth but straight from my heart and soul, "THAT'S UNACCEPTABLE! Get out of my room and don't come back."

That two word phrase, "That's Unacceptable," has stayed etched permanently into my aching brain and has become my internal badge of courage. In that moment I found the courage to say, NO, I cannot and will not accept this. I defy the statistics. I don't care what they say, this is my life and they don't have any right to make predictions for me. In that moment, I made a commitment to myself that win or lose, I will not surrender. I will fight with every fiber of my body and mind to survive. My life was a gift from God and I wasn't going to let anyone or anything take it away without a fight. What I didn't know at the time, was waiting for me just around the corner.

The tumor was diagnosed. Dr. Beyerl sat down to explain to me, Warren, Mom and Dad that my tumor was malignant and not encapsulated as hoped. He was able to remove the definable tumor which I now know is quite remarkable considering the location of the tumor. It was located very deep in the left parietal lobe of the brain and situated near the motor skills.

He paused to allow questions but none came. We all sat in a half circle of chairs facing him, stunned by the word "malignant". Silently I was rationalizing that malignant was O.K. since it had been removed. They cut it out and it was floating somewhere in some pathologist's laboratory. I think I watched too many "doctor" shows as a child.

After the awkward silence, Dr. Beyerl continued. The tumor was very aggressive and was a grade IV malignancy. Malignant brain tumors are graded by two different systems. According to the St. Anne's system, the grading scale goes from one through four with four being the most aggressive malignancies. According to the World Health Organization, grading goes from one through three with three being the most aggressive type tumors.

"What do you call this thing?" I asked, my voice beginning to crack. He wrote it out on a piece of scrap paper and handed it to me. Etched on this tiny insignificant scrap of paper were two words that would change my world forever - glioblastoma multiforme. Anything that awesome sounding had to be intimidating. I tried to pronounce it in my mind. But wait a minute. I had valiantly come through the incredible craniotomy and the surgery was a tremendous success. I felt very good, walking, talking, eating and laughing with staff and friends.

I tried to keep my thoughts positive but Dr. Beyerl, my hero, was not looking very positive. I felt his discomfort. I read between his measured words. I knew this was not good, nor was it over. With one single bound we bypassed the dismal diagnosis, and leaped over to the murky waters of prognosis. More discomfort, more awkward phraseology, all desperately trying NOT to say what had to be said.

The tumor was the most deadly of all brain tumors. There is no known cause, no known cure, and it has a high probability of recurring within a short period of time. Treatments are limited, generally ineffective, and there was little hope of further surgery due to the tumor location. None of this was said directly to me. Again long and agonizing silence, but not being one to beat around the bush, I blurted out the question no one in that room wanted to answer, "How long?" I truly believe that the answer was harder for him than for me and the agonizing seconds when he cleared his throat before answering my tough but insistent question seemed an eternity. I felt sympathy for him as I waited to hear his response but the answer was masterfully disguised under the 'we don't know' clause.

He knew the truth was, the odds were against me. The survival rate for this type of tumor was between 1-2 years. He knew from previous patients, anxious faces mixed with shock and fear, much like our own. He knew from previous conversations, previous outcomes. Being the bearer of such news with a limited ability to offer hope must have left an empty frustration each time it occurred. I could see it pained him deeply and it is only now with some of the same knowledge from my own journey and of others I have grown to love, that I have come to a greater respect for the tough job he has chosen to pursue. The technical expertise must be the easy part. It is no wonder physicians distance themselves from the emotional aspect of their profession.

I felt a twinge of internal resentment because my body had betrayed me. There seemed to be no warning except for those few months I experienced what were medically termed as 'episodes'. They occurred once a month, and weird but true, every time I ate McDonald's or Burger King food. All of a sudden, like a speeding train out of nowhere, I was completely paralyzed for a few seconds. I could hear you, see you and was fully conscious, but I was frozen in motion as if in a panic attack. I had no ability to respond or control it and sometimes would hyper-ventilate. If I could get a sip of water the paralysis disappeared almost instantaneously.

I called my family physician the first time this occurred because it scared me out of my wits. She said it sounded like a hypoglycemic attack and arranged for me to be tested accordingly. The results were positive but I kept insisting this was too weird. No one who had hypoglycemia had the kind of episode that completely terrorized them and sent them into convulsive tears at its conclusion. So I called my doctor's partner to get a second opinion, explaining the bizarre reaction I was having even though I was now working with a recommended nutritionist. He agreed with his partner that it was hypoglycemia, so I concluded, it was my over-reaction to this stressful occurrence. The episodes didn't last long or occur often enough to give them too much further thought, until now.

Even now, doctors cannot say with any certainty that these 'episodes' were seizures as they did not fit the profile but they must have been occurring due to the tumor. I still find it incredible that I intuitively knew these were not normal even though I had medical assurance from several physicians that it was typical. This experience taught me early on to listen to my body first and outside opinions second.

That evening, due to sheer exhaustion, Warren and my family left me to sleep but sleep was not available for me. I called an old friend who had always been a source of comfort. He came at 11:30 p.m. when the whole hospital was quiet. We sat and talked, we sat and cried, we sat and prayed. Finally we laughed. What else can you do when all the bad stuff is said, the tears have been shed, and the petitions have been made? Laugh. Jimmy Buffet sings, "If we couldn't laugh, we'd all go insane." We had a drink (fruit juice) and reminisced about the "old days" when life was simpler.

It was over a week that I had been in the hospital and I had not seen the love and light of my life, my daughter Krystal. It was so hard. I had an 8x11 picture of her by my bed. Nothing made me cry until I looked at her beautiful smiling face and those big brown eyes and I would melt into tears. I could not bear the thought of leaving her. I had not been able to let her see me because I felt I would scare her with my scar and shaven head. It took several days ignoring well meaning people before I could have her come visit me.

In the meantime, she bought me three tams, (those flat hats called berets in France or tams in Scotland) and sent them in for me. The surgeon was very considerate and only shaved a section of my long blonde hair so with the tam on one side, I looked as if nothing even happened. Krystal couldn't wait to come see me. Within seconds, my fears disappeared as this delightful child bounced into my room, onto my bed, and into my arms. She had gotten all dressed up for me. After many hugs and kisses, she leaned over and pulled off the hat. She went around the bed to see my scar, and simply said matter-of-factly, "Boy, did they scalp you!" No big deal. She could handle it. I was energized by her.

I saw in those big brown eyes my reason to fight; to fight for every moment, every ounce of strength, to hold on to any shred of hope, to pray for courage to go on. I determined in my heart, there and then, I was going to dance at her wedding and she can't get married until she's forty. We have since lowered the age to thirty because I want to enjoy my grandchildren as well. I later told Warren that if ever I should falter, he was to hold her in front of my face and remind me that she was my strongest motivation. She has lived up to the role.

Never underestimate the understanding of a child. All the while I was in the hospital and unable to find enough strength to see her, everyone told me she was fine and doing very well. When I saw her I knew and I felt they were wrong. Not intentionally because my daughter has the capacity to make you think everything is O.K. but she cannot fool me just as I cannot fool her. She told me nearly a year later, that she was so hurt that she could not come to the hospital to see me. She thought I did not *want* to see her. How far from the truth, but my actions did not match my feelings. I apologized to her and she accepted my explanation but we have been more open and honest with our feelings ever since I learned how much we needed each other.

It is easy to overlook the needs of a child and the intense feelings they may have especially in time of crisis. Keeping the lines of communication open becomes of utmost importance in letting children express their fears, their anger, the anxiety they may be feeling. Many children take the burdens of these emotions upon themselves, often not knowing how to define or express what they are feeling. Adults, in an effort to protect, often neglect to explain things in terms a child can digest.

Give them no more than they ask for. My daughter's doctor told me to remember the story of the boy who asked his parents, "Where do I come from?" The parents proceed to give a very detailed explanation of the reproduction process after which the little boy says, "I meant what city do I come from." Remember to give them an opportunity to ask whatever they need or want to know. Never lie to protect them. Just give them simple reassurances and simple details. Sometimes it helps to get help from objective sources as one's own emotions can interfere with objectivity.

Remember children do not get cluttered with details as we adults are inclined. We complicate where they simplify. An example of the simplicity with which a child sees things occurred a few weeks after I returned home.

Krystal asked me to make her favorite lunch, macaroni and cheese. I stood looking at her with a blank stare realizing I did not have a clue on how to begin this task I had previously done many times before. Again, she asked, "Mom, could you please make me macaroni and cheese for lunch?" Flustered and somewhat confused, I said, "Honey, I'd love to but Mommy can't remember the recipe." "Oh", she said with understanding, "I guess THAT'S what the doctor took out of your head when you had surgery. Just remember at your next appointment, to ask him where he put the recipe for my macaroni and cheese, please."

After two weeks being confined in the hospital, I was getting anxious on the one hand to get home and be with Warren and Krystal but on the other hand, it was frightening to leave the constant care and supervision of the hospital. It had become a safe haven with its round the clock care. I felt apprehensive about not having a doctor or nurse available. However, it was time to move forward.

Alas, permission was granted to go home.

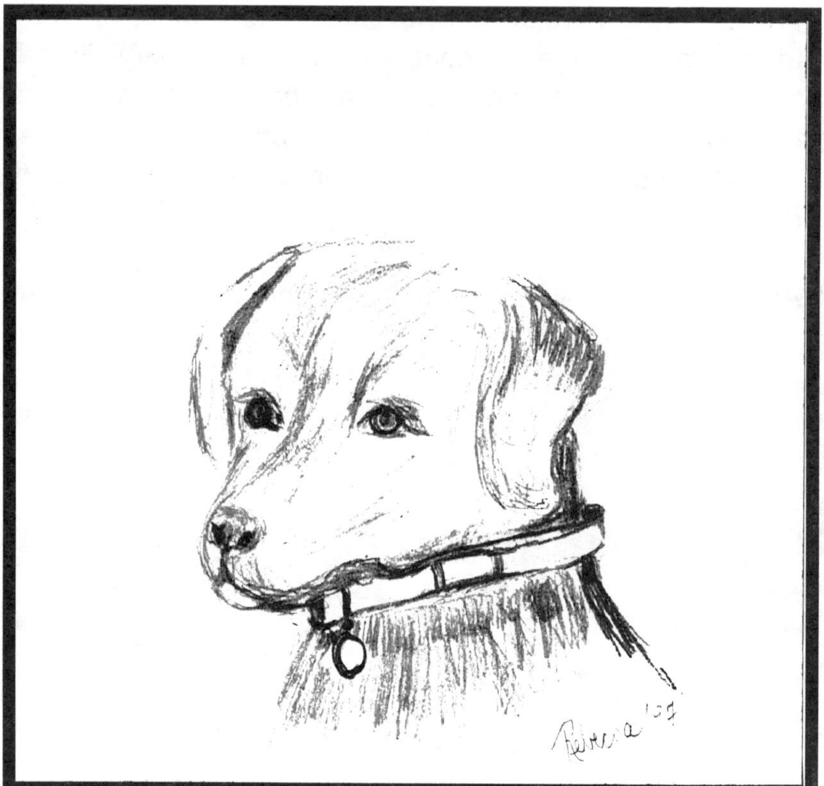

Murphy Brown

No Living in Kansas...
When You've Been to OZ

The day was crisp with the scent of autumn leaves and bright with a warm glowing sun as we walked hand-in-hand up the walkway to my house. The radiant yellow chrysanthemums were in bloom and were a welcome change from the many floral arrangements I received in the hospital. It all looked so beautiful. At once, I began to cry. Warren didn't understand why but in that moment I realized my life, our life, had changed forever. When I walked through the massive arched doorway of my lovely old tudor home, nothing would ever be the same.

Inside I immediately began to relax and the warmth and comfort of home began to lift my spirit. My brother, Brian along with my two brother-in-laws, Mick and John had cleaned the yard, fixed the roof which three previous contractors were unable to correct while my sisters and my mother had cleaned the house, done the laundry, and taken care of the dog. My congregation generously arranged to provide meals for me and my family for over a month. There were many visitors who came to share their concern and love. I am truly blessed to have so many giving people surround me.

During the following month, my Mom, my Dad, my sister, Cindy, and my sister-in-law, Lori had all taken a turn in caring for me, Krystal and Warren. Now it was time to be on our own. Mom and I had been out walking with my 95 pound Labrador Retriever, Murphy Brown, for a few weeks now and I was getting stronger. I knew their departure was imminent and I began to feel anxiety. It was a feeling returning from long ago and I couldn't quite remember why it felt so familiar, that déjà vu feeling like you have been there before. After they packed and got in the car, I watched as they drove away and my mind flashed back thirty-three years earlier with sudden clarity.

When I was five years old, I had a tremendous stomach ache which the doctor told my Mom was merely a virus that would pass in a few days. When a few days passed and I was doubled over in pain, my mother rushed me into the emergency room at the hospital, just in time to find out that my appendix had ruptured and peritonitis (poisoning of the blood) had set in. They said if she had waited another hour, I would have died. I was listed in critical condition for two weeks before they would offer any hope of a recovery.

The memory that suddenly flashed back was the same feeling I had each night when my parents were forced to leave the hospital. I would walk to the elevator with them and kiss them good-bye. I was a brave little five year-old until the doors closed and I was alone. Then I felt an overwhelming fear and ache in the depth of my heart, reaching all the way into the pit of my stomach. I would run to the window in my room and look for them in the parking lot. Tears streamed down my face every time they had to leave. Today, I felt that same overwhelming ache and need to cry.

After weeks ranging from cluttered commotion to utter chaos, the house was now eerily quiet. I had time to think. With each two mile walk I began to think about this prognosis, trying to figure out what to do. One day, in particular, it struck me that I could die. It was kind of a delayed reaction, I admit. It had been weeks since my brain learned of the prognosis we were facing. But today, my heart heard it for the first time.

Murphy and I burst through the front door and I plunged to the floor pounding the carpet with my fists, screaming and yelling until I could yell no more, choked from hoarseness. All my emotions came from my very center like an erupting volcano. The heated fury poured out of me like lava bursting from a mountain of fear and anger. Murphy ran into hiding as I kicked the hall carpet in rage, like a child having a tantrum, and after crying and sobbing and releasing all the rage and anger and fear I felt inside, I pleaded with my God for my life. I begged for strength to endure pain, for wisdom to make intelligent decisions on treatments, for power to pull myself up and to encourage others and, finally, for time to accomplish my goals.

I never asked the age old question, "Why me?" I wanted to know, "Why anyone?" This disease makes no sense. It does not distinguish. It takes young, old, healthy, strong, fit and productive humans and touches the very core of life and being.

It reaches into the caverns unreachable for centuries by medicine, and threatens the essence of who you are. You cannot prevent it by not smoking, by eating healthy, by medication or lifestyle. My thoughts were racing. How do you stop your body from producing these run-away cells? A Glioblastoma, I thought, was like a speeding train without a conductor to direct its path. It was on a collision course with my very self and you barely had time to think. If ever there was a need for Superman to step in front of this run-away menace, it certainly was now. But there I was alone, having to find that person deep within myself.

I called the American Brain Tumor Association and requested the literature specific to my tumor. My family circumvented it from getting to me as they figured I couldn't handle it. Even the telephone operator asked me if I wanted the prognosis information since many previous patients had not wanted to know such statistical data. My sincere response was, "Well, I have a glioblastoma, I think I NEED to know what I am dealing with here!"

Being persistent, I requested it again and got what I asked for, although perhaps more than I bargained for: the prepared pamphlet indicated only 1% survive 5 years and less than 1% survive longer. Most survive 1-2 years. I stared at the bleak numbers in complete horror.

There was no one around at that moment and I closed my eyes and laid my head on the kitchen table. It was worse than even I could have imagined. Even AIDS gave people more time than this little pamphlet held out for me. I thought of my husband and realized how stoic he had been, knowing this painful information from the near beginning and dreading its possible outcome and yet always maintaining a positive and hopeful outlook for me. It must have been unbearable for him to feel so helpless against something so intangible, invisible, and seemingly so invincible.

This is cancer... cancer of the brain. Somehow that simple yet potent fact had never dawned on me in the hospital when they said "malignancy". After reading the brochure from the ABTA over several times, I became quite aware of just how devastating this disease is and how hard it would be to fight it. It looked so hopeless, so insurmountable.

Just when it seemed I had finally found everything in my life that made me happy; a great husband, a beautiful daughter, terrific parents, supportive and loving family and friends, a fabulous new career, someone hit the brake switch and it all came to a screeching halt. An unwelcome "alien" had entered my very being, threatening my ability to defend my deepest thoughts, torching my heart with fear, and devouring my very soul. It lurked in the dark caverns of my brain, trying to take away my mind and my will.

Perhaps we all face a certain denial about our mortality. When you have youth and health, you may know someday you will die, but you never really think about the consequences. You accept it as a part of life, the final curtain, all good things must come to an end.

But not until you are ready, somehow you reason. Here I was looking up at a curtain the medical establishment had assured me would drop quickly on "my show".

Could I accept this? Would I? The day was too beautiful. The world with all its troubles was still a compelling place to be, and life with all its dysfunction was still too precious to let go.

I took many walks along the same path day after day, but with many different thoughts. In particular, I was deeply affected by an audio taped presentation. I listened over and over to the message given by a minister I would later meet in my travels. He talked about never losing heart and some insight into living a long life. He told of an old man who was approached with the question of how he managed to live so long. The old man said, "Do you really want to know how to live a long life?" "Yes, please tell me", was the reply. With a deep, slow, deliberate voice, the old man said, "Just don't die". How sweetly simple I thought with a sudden smile. Just don't die. That became my plan - kind of like a reverse of the Nike plan for fitness.

There are No Simple Solutions ... Only Intelligent Choices

My perspective of life was altered permanently but it was for the better. So many things became quite insignificant, others took on greater significance. Life is a gift, and I intended to do everything necessary to preserve it.

Precious little things took on great significance. When you are able to breathe in the fresh air, absorb the clear blue sky, roll in the green earth beneath your feet; when you can smell the roses literally and figuratively, and sing songs of birds and children, life takes on a sweetness not tasted before. When you can be there to pick up your child from school and help with homework, when walking the dog is a pleasure and not a chore, when holding a baby kitten brings out the mother instinct, life takes on special meaning with each and every breath. I was never so aware of the sensory pleasures of life as when it was threatened to be taken away.

There was also a new found sense of responsibility for my future. I knew if it was to "be", it was going to be up to me to search and research, and read and scour and process and ask the right questions. I was not going to wait around for someone else to determine my next move so I began reading everything I could get my hands on. Books about brain tumors and what to expect were few and far between to put it mildly, but books about healing, remarkable recoveries, mind and body connection, cancer, et cetera, were abundant and I absorbed and literally devoured information.

The information began to mold my sense of self: my knowledge became empowering, my direction became clear. I developed a sort of healing "map" which led me down many paths and surprisingly created that "light at the end of the tunnel" that we all seem to search for during crisis. Sometimes, it felt like it might be the light of an on-coming train, as they say, but there was light all the same. And with each new day there was renewed hope, renewed determination.

My education was just beginning. All my life I have battled with maintaining my ideal weight. I needed to work out excessively to maintain a reasonable weight and watch every morsel of food to prevent gaining. I had always eaten a healthy balanced diet, but the year prior to my diagnosis, I had suffered two miscarriages and retained weight from the ensuing stress and grief. At a height of merely five-foot four-inches (and that is stretching it) I was not prepared for what followed.

After brain surgery, Decadron is a common drug prescribed to minimize swelling. Someone, however, forgot to tell me that Decadron is a steroidal drug which not only creates a sense of well-being but also stimulates an incredible appetite and subsequent sudden weight gain. Thanks guys for overlooking this small detail until I gained fifty pounds in two months! Not only did the weight gain distort my appearance, but the steroids (Decadron) also cause what is called affectionately in the industry, the 'moon face'. To be more specific, my face swelled up like a casaba melon. I could barely see my eyes. That was an understatement as I hardly recognized myself. I have a theory, quite unscientific, but I think Decadron reduces the swelling in your brain by transferring it directly to your cheeks (choose whichever you use least). Of course, that is not medically proven ... yet.

With my hair partially shaven, my face swollen beyond my own recognition, and my body overwhelmed with an additional fifty pounds, it was all I could do to maintain my self esteem. The logical me kept repeating in my head, 'stop complaining, at least you are alive' but one quick glance in the mirror could set the emotional me off on a crying jag for hours.

Even with makeup and on a good day, I looked like the Pillsbury Dough Boy with a bad hair cut. The biggest 'ouch' came when I stopped in at my office to pick up some paperwork and a co-worker did not even recognize me and asked if I needed help. My mind said, 'I guess I must need help if you don't even know who I am' but my mouth just fell open unable to make an audible sound. I felt lost inside myself. At that point in time, I was.

Logically, my solution was to simply get off the nasty stuff - with side effects like these who needs it? Not so easy, as your body creates a quick attachment and goes through painful withdrawal as you wean yourself off these wonder drugs. Gradually, I eased off the steroids, using a prescribed dose for one day, half the next day, following that routine for a week to allow my body to adjust to the lower dose. The following week, I would again cut the dose for every other day, and so on until finally none.

This was a painful process. My body had become dependent on the steroids to minimize pain. As I weaned off the drug, my legs and joints would ache, my head would pound, my stomach would wrench. Warren would have to wake up in the middle of the night to help me out of bed and walk me to the bathroom. In the early morning it would take twenty minutes to get down the stairs, with my back to the wall just in case a leg would give out. Sometimes I would just sit down and go down the stairs on my butt. Sometimes the pain was so intense I was forced, against even my strongest will, to increase the steroid dose until another day. My determination eventually became stronger than the drug, but there were days I thought I would never win the battle.

Dilantin is also commonly prescribed as an anti-seizure medication which I began taking in the hospital. It gave me a strange "burning sensation" over my body but I didn't pay much attention at that time. However, after a few weeks at home, I developed an allergic reaction to Dilantin. My entire body was covered with incredibly huge itchy welts. After six weeks at home, I woke one morning itching and burning all over. I had a rash on my chest that looked like a severe sun burn. Within hours, my entire body looked like I had been in the sun for days.

Aveeno baths in cold water, every anti-itch cream known to man and pharmacy, tepid tea baths, all did little to ease the agony of the itch "witch". She tortured me for weeks. I scratched until my skin was raw. The half life of Dilantin is rather long, which means it stays in your system for a while. So there was no relief for many weeks even though I had been switched to Phenobarbital, used as an anti-seizure medication. I continue to use phenobarbital to prevent seizure activity which could occur from a tumor recurrence, scar tissue from surgery, disrupted tissue, etc.

The journey many describe as the "roller coaster ride from hell" had only just begun. It became increasingly necessary to "roll with the punches" as this roller coaster takes you up and down with sudden unexpected curves and jolts that turn your life completely upside down at times. It was at this point that I began my search for the next step. I was advised to start radiation treatment by the radiologist and to begin a high dose chemotherapy program with stem cell rescue by the oncologist. Both seemed to demand my attention and decisions immediately. I knew there was a sense of urgency, but I needed some time to evaluate my choices and options.

The radiologist patiently described the method of standard beam radiation he recommended. It was a very precisely focused beam, three beams in my case, that are aimed at a very small "window" mapped out through the computer. The radiation's purpose was to zap any cells which may be remaining after surgery. I was encouraged to begin as soon as possible before any cells became active.

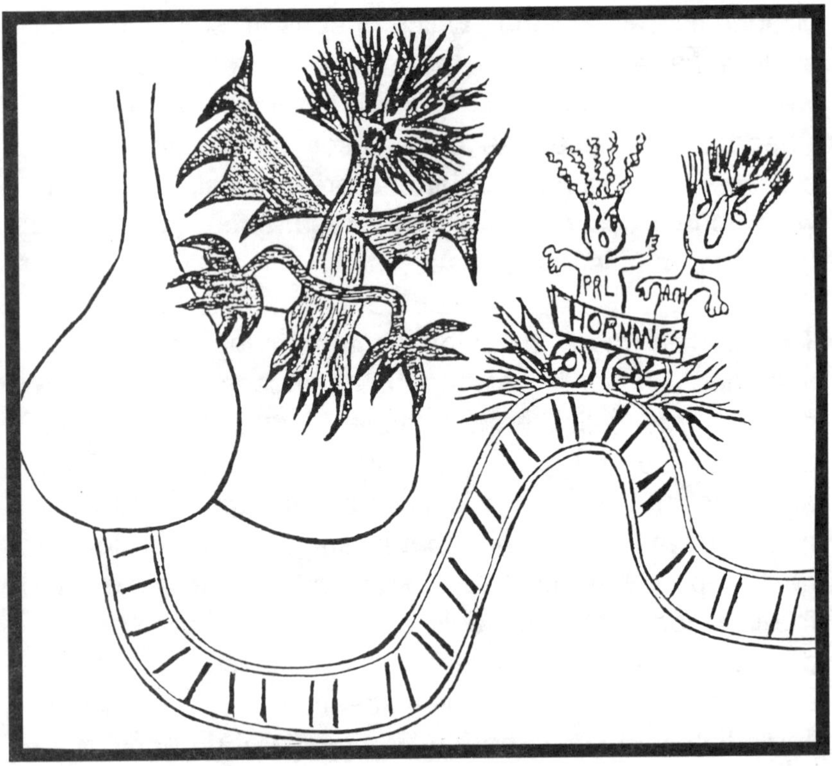

Runaway Hormones
Life With A Pituitary Adenoma

by Sonia Scott

The oncologist and his specialty were a mystery to me. Chemotherapy was as foreign to me as the Foreign Legion. I never knew anyone who had chemotherapy treatments or if I did, they never discussed it with me. I did not even know what they were talking about, wondering does it come in gel caps or is it a disgusting tasting liquid. I am a real baby when it comes to taking medicines so the thought of this chilled me to the bone.

As it happened, I did know someone who was familiar with chemotherapy. Warren's Aunt Irene had recently been diagnosed with breast cancer and she was so kind and helpful as she explained to me that chemotherapy was treatment using chemotherapeutic drugs. Some drugs could be taken intravenously through a vein, some could be injected intra-muscularly into fatty tissue or muscle where it is absorbed by the system, and some could be swallowed in pill form. It was a simple and concise and a clear explanation, sufficient for my needs at the time.

The oncologist was young and pleasant. He explained a desire to take an aggressive approach due to my young age. As the second overall largest cause of death in older Americans, doctors were accustomed to seeing brain tumors in patients in their sixties and seventies. In recent years this deadly disease has increased in a much younger population, many in their thirties and forties. Brain cancer has also become the second largest cause of cancer death in children under the age of fifteen.

So when the oncologist suggested a new and aggressive approach to chemotherapy, it certainly made sense to me. He began talking about stem cell harvesting and high dose chemo-therapeutic agents called Carboplatin and Cisplatin. Again, I felt overwhelmed with an urgency to make a decision while what I was only hearing was blah, blah, stem cell (what's a stem cell?) blah blah blah (how do you harvest one?) blah blah blah...

The process was still in trial phases and it was not certain of the success rate. The procedure involves taking out healthy blood and siphoning, so to speak, the healthy stem cells which would later mature into healthy blood cells. These are stored while your body receives a high dose of very toxic but hopefully effective drugs, such as Cisplatin and Carboplatin. To minimize the damage to the immune system, the "harvested" stem cells are then returned to the body to restore itself. The advance of modern technology was overwhelming in its implications. It sounded sensible but I had some reservations.

Time out for a second opinion. Fortunately my mother-in-law knew someone who got me an appointment at Memorial Sloan-Kettering, one of the largest cancer centers in the world. MSK called me the day I got home from the hospital after surgery to schedule an appointment immediately. I was impressed with their efficiency but I silently was resenting that I had to go to the largest cancer center in the world at all.

Another adventure? Well, we decided to make it one. I don't know how else I would have gotten through everything if it was not for the many friends who held out their hands and hearts for me, Warren and Krystal to hold. Sharon and I had been friends from our teens, a life in New Hampshire that seems like centuries ago. She sent a hand-written note offering us another pair of eyes and ears to take along on our conference with the medical professionals at Sloan-Kettering. With her keen ability to ask questions, Warren and I were able to listen better and absorb the answers. Sharon and I took copious notes which we compared later in the car ride home.

We were immediately ushered into the hustle and bustle of this busy medical mammoth. I was instantly struck by the size of the buildings that made up Memorial Sloan-Kettering Cancer Center, towering over its 1275 York Avenue address in Manhattan. Realizing that every floor was dedicated to one type of cancer or another, seeing the waiting lines of patients to be admitted, I shuddered to think of the reason I was there.

Admitted promptly, we were directed to the Neuro-oncology floor. After an extensive examination by an internist who seemed to be amazed that I had just been through surgery for a Glioblastoma brain tumor, a team of five doctors crowded into the tiny examining room. The three of us were seated, they each took positions juxtaposed against the unused walls and doorways.

Sitting across from Warren, up on the examining table, my legs were swinging back and forth with anxiety. Sharon readied her note pad and our collective questions. I immediately gravitated to Dr. Mark Malkin, who seemed to have the lead in the discussion. His manner was instantly kind and direct. He and his colleagues were genuinely impressed with my positive recovery from surgery.

After the appropriate introductions, I began with my agenda of questions; how many people do you treat a year for this, how long have you been in this field, how many are you currently treating, how soon must we determine a course of action, what are my options, are you familiar with the stem cell harvest program?

There was a calmness about this team of highly trained professionals but we all agreed later that more importantly was the sincere feeling of care and concern for my well-being and the quality of life I wanted to maintain. This took precedence over the direction of conversation.

Dr. Malkin seemed to know what we needed to hear and he elaborated on the details so I became comfortable with the answers. We discussed the proposed chemotherapy using the blood stem cell rescue or sometimes called "harvest". Dr. Malkin explained it had been conducted as a clinical trial.

Dr. Malkin was straight with me and answered every single question. New Jersey has a company that advertises, 'an educated consumer is the best customer' and having subscribed to that philosophy for many years, I was keenly interested in knowing everything possible about this tumor. My questions were not easy for Dr. Malkin because I wanted to know details and an immediate, preferably positive, outcome to the facts I assimilated. I recall my husband being horrified when he read my notes, after asking Dr. Malkin to explain to me what happens when you die. I know it seems macabre to ask for details when your focus is on NOT needing that information, but I found comfort in simply knowing it was not necessarily painful. I will not elaborate on details as everyone's interest may differ and each doctor's explanation may differ.

What was keenly important to me was that Dr. Malkin was willing to tell me the best possible answer to what I felt was important to know and never told me I didn't need to know this or that.

He was professional, honest, and suggested it might be easier to obtain the treatment in New Jersey as opposed to schlepping back and forth to New York City. I agreed that I would like to conserve my strength for other activities.

He and the rest of the team were not promoting the stem cell rescue treatment as they were concerned about the toxicity of the drugs and the effect on the quality of life issues. I was relieved to learn of their experience, since the trials were going on for three years and the results were discouraging. Right then and there I knew that was not the treatment we had hoped to find.

We left Memorial Sloan-Kettering and decided to walk a few blocks to a cozy Italian restaurant to discuss our thoughts about the morning conference. It was raining and as we quickly crossed the street, my mind was on the earlier discussion. Sharon suddenly grabbed my arm and pulled me out of the way of a speeding New York City taxi-cab. We joked that my odds of getting run over by a New York cabby were probably higher than that of getting a brain tumor.

Lunch was delicious and I indulged myself with one glass of red wine. We all agreed the doctors were excellent and we returned home feeling closer to an intelligent decision.

Dr. Malkin was the first physician that truly inspired hope in me and I wanted him to know it. When I initially met with him, and later on the telephone, I begged him and his associates to tell me someone, anyone, had actually made it beyond five years since that was the farthest extent on the statistical charts. They were reticent to make any clear cut statements at first but I persisted. Finally, they said, 'Yes, some three, some five, and a very few even ten years' and HOPE was born! I clung to that single thin thread. I didn't want or really need details. I just knew in my heart that if someone else could do it, so could I.

We made a decision not to pursue the high dose chemotherapy at that time as I felt it was too toxic for me. I know my body is extremely sensitive to any medications. My doctors used to tell me they had to prescribe pediatric doses for me to avoid negative reactions. As much as I needed the best treatment, I wanted to find a balance between the strength of medication and the strength of the body's own immune system.

We considered Brachy-therapy, which involves the inserting of tiny radioactive pellets into the tumor site to blast away the outer perimeter of where the tumor was located. However, my tumor was not the appropriate shape for this procedure. Dr. Malkin made me laugh when he said it was shaped like a dumb-bell and therefore not a good site for this procedure. He could have said an hour glass but no, a dumb-bell summed it up completely!

Being duly impressed with the caring approach I received at Memorial Sloan-Kettering, I returned home with my decision to begin radiation therapy as my initial treatment. Medical technology has rapidly progressed in three years and now the time and methods used for radiation vary. As research continues, medical advances will no doubt improve the techniques and timing of radiation modalities.

With the decision in hand, I begged Warren to take me away for a few days before I began the treatment. I wanted him to take me to our favorite place in Maine, the little town of Ogunquit. Its name means "Beautiful Place by the Sea" and it couldn't be more so. We had found this place eleven years ago when we were first married and we loved it so much we returned every year on our anniversary or in the autumn season. I was sure it would be therapeutic with its rocky coastline, its quaint artsy little town in Perkins Cove, and of course, the one mile walk known as The Marginal Way, a winding, wielding path along the rocks and cliffs overlooking the powerful Atlantic Ocean.

Warren worried that the setting with all our happy memories might make me maudlin. To the contrary, I never felt so invigorated. The air was sun-laden but crisply fall. The feisty ocean thrashed its white crested waves against the rocky crevices of the New England shoreline. You could taste its saltiness in the biting air.

Warren and Krystal walked out on the rocks together and I was filled with awe of this wonderful man who cared for me and our daughter with the same determination of the waves crashing nearby. His strength would lift me up, his stubborn determination would not let me falter, his hand in mine guided me through the darkest moments, and with him I felt safe. I remember the reason I married him was he made me feel safe.

His unconditional love reinforced my own faith. Knowing we were in this together and we would fight together gave me strength. Our love would be tested by this great monster, our relationship would be challenged in ways we would only learn later, our lives would be changed in ways we could not fathom at that early point, but we had each other and we had a deep love and respect for each other that would raise us up over any mountains we would encounter.

If there was such thing as human glue, it would be personified by our little Krystal Lee. At seven years old, she had been my constant companion and a delightful child. She had an attachment to me and I to her, that some implied was not "healthy". My response was that our bond was "heavenly" because it filled the spiritual, physical, mental and emotional needs of our "family".

Our brief weekend in Maine was more therapeutic than any drug I could have ever found. We stood huddled together, all three of us in the white gazebo overlooking the ocean and curving coastline. For a few moments we were transported beyond the tumor and its pressing weight on our minds. On our last night, we dressed to the 'max' and dined at our favorite restaurant in Maine,

The Clay Hill Farm. It is a long drive down an old dusty country road, situated out in the middle of nowhere. It is the kind of road that makes you wonder 'who in their right mind would put a restaurant way out here?' Suddenly, through the velvety black sky of the nippy New England night, we see the twinkling lights outlining the trees surrounding the magnificent old farm house. It has been converted to an elegant dining experience. After leaving our car with the valet, we are greeted by the playing of the Grand Piano.

Krystal wore a blue taffeta party dress with straps over her bare delicate shoulders. I curled her long brown hair into voluminous locks and painted her nails, quite a victory since my right arm was still somewhat dyslexic from surgery. We had to search the country stores of Maine to find her first pair of nylon stockings for the evening event. I wore a black velvet jacket trimmed with gold over a white silk blouse and a black velvet skirt. My blonde hair was still long on one side and with the black tam Krystal had given me at the hospital, we took pictures, forgetting just for the moment that anything at all was wrong in our lives.

We dined on exquisite rack of lamb, lobster, and seafood. We sent Krystal to the piano with dollar bills and a request for our wedding song, "Love Lifts Us Up Where We Belong".

We came back to New Jersey with Maine's motto "The Way Life Should Be", amply prepared to face the challenging treatment ahead with the same motto.

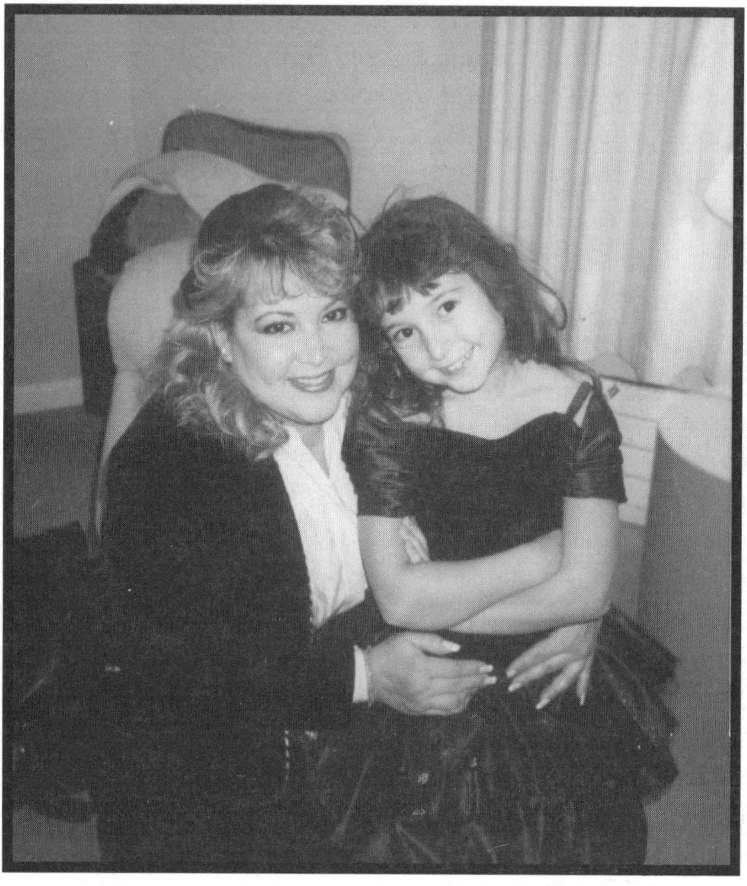

An Evening at The Clay Hill Farm
Ogunquit, Maine

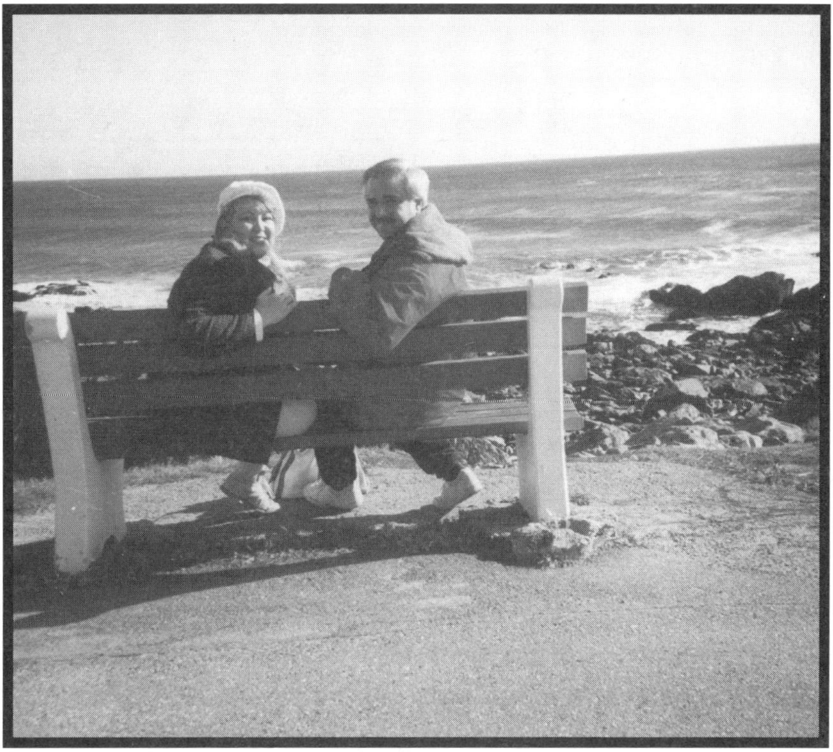

"Love Lifts Us Up"
Warren and Rebecca

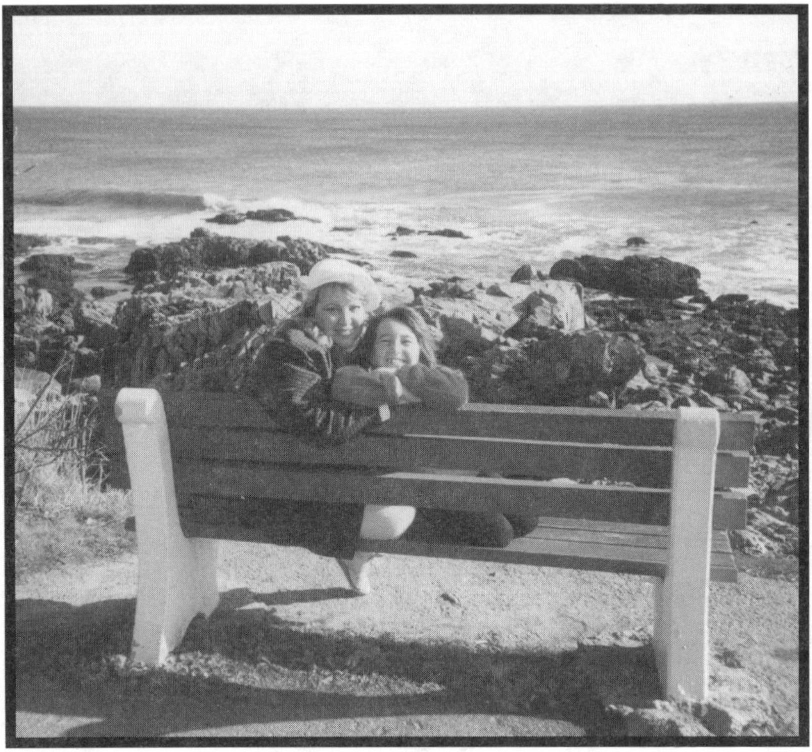

Maine - "The Way Life Should Be"

Open Mouth, Insert Foot
Radiation Treatment

I managed to by-pass the doctor who gave me his negative, albeit "facts only" attitude, and met with his partner. Dr. Schwartz was compassionate, kind and gentle as well as informative and non-threatening in his evaluation of time. I had many questions which were answered with reassurance and confidence. His honesty about the unknown was balanced with knowledge gained through experience in this field.

Dr. Schwartz willingly shared his expertise and knowledge with me before I agreed to proceed with the therapy. He explained that radiation therapy had evolved from whole brain radiation which often caused serious brain damage to the current, more precise method, which directed the radiation beams to a very small area or "window" at the tumor site, thus sparing healthy brain tissue. He would use a 6 Million Volt Linear Accelerator, localized to the tumor site and a very small margin of surrounding tissue. I would receive approximately 6,000 centiGray (cGy) or rads directed at the imperceptible roots of the tumor.

Carefully, he explained the possible side effects of standard beam radiation such as edema, swelling of tissue, ringing in the ears, loss of hair, scarring of brain tissue, along with headaches from the swelling tissue, a possible sunburned look, and a 1% chance of brain damage. Even a 1% chance of brain damage rattled me but he again kindly reassured me that the chances were minimal.

Although I desperately wanted to get off the steroids completely, Dr. Schwartz recommended that I not reduce the amount below eight milligrams. However, due to the pressure of the new treatment and its unknown effects, I decided to maintain my dosage of Decadron at twelve milligrams.

His staff was fabulous with preparing my head for treatment using a procedure called brain mapping. Using a CT scanner, the site to be radiated is set up via a simulation computer. The radiation technicians were so careful to align everything accurately that it took hours of laying there motionless while several staff members as well as the doctor checked and re-checked. Dr. Schwartz explained that the goal was to reach the tumor site from several angles with minimal damage to the healthy cells and brain tissue. Radiation was necessary despite the fact that the tumor was successfully removed. There are tiny microscopic cells which remain undetected or unresolvable by surgery alone. These cells must be eliminated so as not to cause a recurrence somewhere down the road. I would receive a total of 6020 rads of standard beam radiation over a seven week duration.

Being intrepid about more pain and side effects, it was a great relief to find that this treatment is quite painless. It is not without its side effects, both long term and short term, but it is a relatively painless procedure. You lay comfortably on a table and in a few seconds a beam of invisible light is flashed at the tumor site. The hardest part is laying motionless while the "brain beam" does its 'magic'.

I wanted to be sure that the 1% chance of damage did not occur so I recited things in my head during the "zapping" time. I started with songs and would try to get all the verses correct before the "beamer" stopped. I decided to memorize the books of the Bible in order from Genesis to Revelation and try to recite them mentally each time I went for radiation. By the end of my treatment, I was able to recite all sixty-six books of the Old and New Testament without a single mistake. A few months later, a visiting minister asked my congregation who was able to recite all the books of the Bible and I was proud to be the first brain tumor patient to raise my hand very high.

Positive thinking and imagery can produce powerful results. Some of my friends said they imagined the beam as warm sunshine washing over them, others thought about soldiers with little swords doing battle with the "bad" cells. My good friends, Flo and Henry and their daughter, Nicole came up with the greatest idea. Flo drew a picture of her brain with the tumor in pencil. She placed it on her refrigerator. Then every night before going to bed, she and her husband and daughter would take turns lightly erasing the tumor area. I have a very strong feeling that picture will portray real life. There is

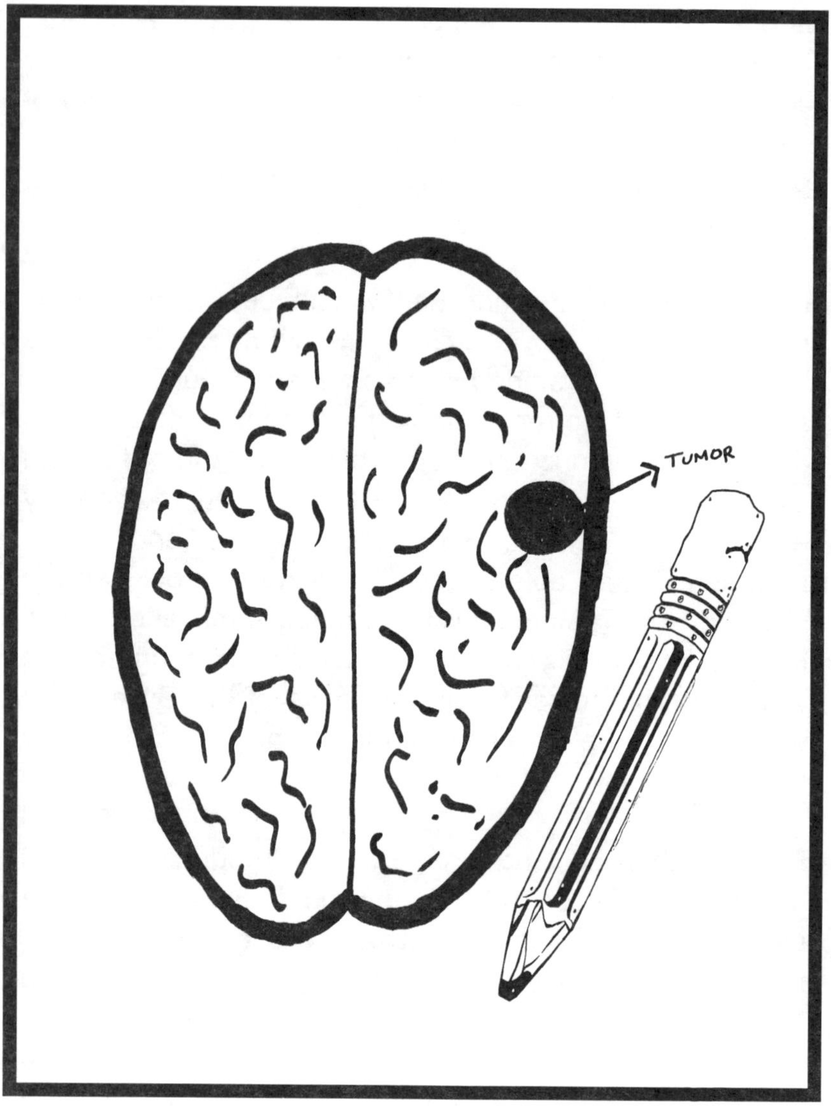

Flo's Brain
The Disappearing Tumor
by Flo Marazia

such positive reinforcement and yet it is open and honest in recognizing there is a consistent effort required to 'erase' the tumor permanently.

Flo, who is also a survivor of an astrocytoma Grade III, with a genuinely positive attitude, finds my form of visualization somewhat entertaining. I admit it takes some chutzpah but I swear it has worked for me. After several MRI scans came back with what was called areas of 'white enhancement' and later 'spots or foci', I became aggravated by the uncertainty of what it might be. THEY said, "It could be tumor cells, it could be scar tissue, it could be disrupted brain tissue."

I decided the old craniotomy needed some housekeeping. These spots had to go - so every time I took a shower, and that can be two or three times a day, I would sing to the melody from the movie musical, South Pacific. The younger generation probably will have no idea what I am talking about, but I would sing, "I'm gonna wash these spots right out of my head, I'm gonna wash these spots right out of my head, I'm gonna wash these cells right out of my brain, and send them down the drain" using the tune Mitzi Gaynor made popular in the sixties. It may have something to do with my love of water and showers or a frustrated desire to sing Broadway tunes, but after several months of singing those spots down the drain, even my surgeon was inclined to admit there were significantly fewer spots on my scans. Weird science or incredible mind/body connection? Does it really matter? It worked.

I recently applied the same technique and the same tune on some aggravating and persistent plantar warts, just changing the words to suit the current need. I have tried every medical remedy now for over a year to no avail, but in a matter of weeks of singing and focusing on eradicating the warts, even I was surprised to find them peeling off with healthy pink skin underneath. Who would have thought it possible? Actually, my daughter's pediatrician shared that secret with her when she had warts. He told her she could will away the warts and that Mommy could do the same with her tumor. I'll admit at the time it sounded like wishful thinking, but I figured, wishful thinking was a cousin to positive thinking and what could it hurt to try?

While I used memorization techniques and old broadway tunes to accomplish my purpose, others have used visualization to accomplish theirs, but hey, whatever works for you. The point is to approach this therapy as well as any other with the utmost belief that it is going to work for you. If your mind believes it, your body has a better chance of getting the message and following directions.

It is my conviction that the body has been intelligently designed to heal itself. Sometimes we have to get it on the right track, but with a little gentle redirecting, it can often do wonders for us in return.

Knowledge is empowering and enables you to take some control of a situation which seems to be uncontrollable. While knowledge is not a cure, it may be critical to your finding what you need and what is best for you. Today, technology is on the brink of some amazing and exciting break through treatments. The advances being made in neuro-science hold promise for the first time in many years. New methods of delivering radiation, such as the gamma-knife and radio-surgery, are evidence that we each must continue our survival education.

A recent approval of the Gliadel wafers seems to offer hope for a better delivery system for chemotherapy needed to reach brain tumor sites. These biodegradable wafers are implanted at the tumor site at the time of surgery, thereby eliminating the exposure of healthy brain tissue to damage and sending an intensified dose of the chemo-therapeutic agent to a specific location in the brain.

The blood-brain barrier is no longer an issue with this treatment. For many years doctors have had to wrestle with the incredible body design that was created with a natural barrier between the body and the brain, known as the blood-brain barrier. This natural and protective defense mechanism often kept brain treatment agents from actually reaching the brain effectively. With the approval of these new wafers, one more hurdle has been made by medical science that may improve the efficacy of chemotherapy for brain tumors and central nervous system tumors.

Be kind to yourself in the education process. Realize that you are being required to learn, in perhaps weeks or months, information it has taken the medical field in its entirety over a century to learn. Give yourself a pat on the back for being able to pronounce some of the foreign terms you have learned and give your brain credit for making new creases in the gray matter to accommodate your new found knowledge. Specialize in your tumor, get to know what is necessary to survive it. Your brain is incredible and you are incredible. Make the most of both.

During my first few treatments, my head was marked with purple "X's" to identify the alignment of my head with the radiation beams. Brilliant as they were, they taped over these marks and told me not to get them wet or we would need to go through the whole alignment process again. Well, duh! This was to go on for seven weeks - how was I suppose to manage not to get them wet especially considering the intense sweating that was occurring as I worried about getting them wet. Dr. Scwartz's partner made a very quiet but useful suggestion - tattoos. This doctor, whom I had previously banished from my room, had come up with the perfect solution to my current dilemma.

Three tiny dots were tattooed at the precise points where radiation was to be directed. After all was said and done, I was grateful for the solution which enabled me to wash my hair during my treatment. In retrospect, I wish I had asked if they could have monogrammed each side of my head with my initials. But, I still have a tiny pin size dot on my forehead that reminds me to be humble whenever I am going to banish someone from my presence. You never know when you may need their help.

If We Couldn't Laugh ...

As I embarked on the Radiation Route, I was determined that it would work. I was determined to keep a positive attitude, always trying to enlist the experts working in this serious environment to laugh with me. I truly believe in the power of laughter and a positive attitude and even more so since reading Norman Vincent Peale's book, "The Power of Positive Thinking", Norman Cousins book, "Anatomy of an Illness", and Bernie Siegel's book, "Love, Medicine and Miracles" as well as "How to Live Between Office Visits".

Much to my husband's dismay, I am also known to quote verses from Jimmy Buffet songs. At this juncture in the journey my favorite verse was, "If we couldn't laugh, we'd all go insane." I decided whatever time I had, I would laugh as often and as much as I could and I haven't gone insane yet although I might admit to coming close a few times. It is my hope to someday meet this hero of the Manatees and let him know he played a part in my recovery.

At about the 5th week of radiation, Dr. Schwartz came in while I was being set up and quite nonchalantly announced, "You're at the point where your hair will start to fall out. It surprised me that he was so matter of fact and that he could pin-point the precise amount of radiation which would cause the fall out. I really didn't buy the idea at first, but prepared myself mentally and emotionally for the possibility.

I felt that in the grand scheme of things, really, what did it matter if I lost all my hair? So when combing my hair one afternoon, I pulled my brush forward, only to see it filled with clumps of what was left of my long blonde hair. It looked like a Chia Pet on a Brush and of course, my inclination was to laugh hysterically. My husband said I had a sick sense of humor, but would he prefer I cry?! I don't think so.

All the losing of hair due to radiation or chemo was highly over-rated to me in any case. Come on, losing my hair was the least of my concerns! So with the help of my friend, Diane, I had it all cut off so we could start over fresh. We actually had a lot of fun and I accentuated my look with big earrings, make-up and humor, and admittedly, some tears. I think it is OK to cry over the loss of anything. I cry over the loss of my tulips, why not my hair? But I also don't get overly concerned for in the spring they do return, as did my hair.

I had been advised by several medical staff personnel to get a wig. Together with my long-time reliable friend, Robin, who for years has advised me on my looks, and my friend Diane, a former hairdresser at Saks Fifth Avenue, we went to a lovely shop with lovely people who deal with many cancer patients and came out with a lovely wig with a lovely price tag of $1,250.00. US dollars, folks. The wig was 50% human hair, eek, and 50% synthetic because I couldn't afford the 100% human hair for $3,000. That could feed a few hungry children, I am sure.

As they say, hind sight is 20/20 vision, and looking back on the fiasco, I can now see how vulnerable I was at that time. I was overwhelmed with what I had been told and not knowing what to expect, left me as the perfect victim. I feel victimized now; now knowing that such an expense was absurd and now knowing that without hair on my head, there was nothing with which to anchor this heavy mop to my scalp. There was more hair in this wig than I had ever had in my entire lifetime. I felt ridiculous.

When I saw my reflection in a store window and my bangs continued to grow shorter and shorter (the wig was slipping off the back) I made an executive decision. I easily pulled it off in the car, put it on the gear shift, and left it there to remind me never to let anyone pressure me about anything again. My baseball cap collection was all I needed. I bought one that said "Bad Hair Day" on it and I was all set thereafter.

In today's celebrity circles, loss of hair or no hair at all seems to be a trademark, thanks to the Demi Moores, Sinaid O'Connors, and Susan Powters of the world. I think I was very in vogue. Several weeks after I got used to this new look, although I wished I had the body to go with it, I was happy to have a funky excuse to call my own. My friend Robin and I went out for dinner and for the first time I took off my hat during dinner. It was so liberating. Some people stared, some pretended not to stare, and others truly never even noticed. The best compliment came from some of my daughter's school-mates who said I was "cool".

Deciding that it took me thirty-eight years to get my hair to the length I wanted, I would take another thirty-eight to grow it back! When it grew in after about a year, it was very dark and curly but weirdly curly only in the radiated sections. The rest remained poker straight. I went with the new look for a while as everyone told me how good it looked. One day I sat at the mirror and knew they were lying so I made an appointment and went to Joanne, my hairdresser, for a very very blonde highlighting. I was born to be a blonde but nature was color blind. With Joanne's expertise, I was able to find myself again, and yes, we do have more fun :).

I was determined that my hair would grow back but I know many brain tumor survivors whose hair did not return completely. We (those of us in the brain tumor circles) say it is much like real estate, location, location, location. The location of the tumor may cause many different effects and outcomes. Try not to take it personally. If my hair did not grow back, I would have just figured some way to deal with it as have my other courageous and ingenious friends.

I was willing and, fortunately, able to drive myself back and forth to the hospital every day for the seven week duration. The most notable side-effect of radiation is the tired weakness you increasingly feel after each subsequent treatment. Your body feels drained of all its energy and quite frankly, it is. I took the attitude that all my energy was being beamed into healing my brain. It took all my mental and physical strength. It is a time to know your resources are needed for a specific assignment and allow your body the time it needs to rest and recover. I have seen some people so anxious to go back to work, they work right through their treatments, but it usually takes its toll on the system. If you have to be treated with subsequent chemotherapy, you will need all the strength you can maintain.

It is only my opinion, but if you don't HAVE to work, then don't. Your body cannot meet every demand placed on it without some consequence. While it may be necessary for some, due to financial constraints, this is a time to re-evaluate priorities and make adjustments. I helped my office by telephone conference and if someone wanted to come by with a file, but I refused to go to the office to work, knowing that it took too much precious energy.

I arranged to go for the radiation therapy early in the day, so I could take a nap before having to pick up Krystal from school. However, my neighbor, Linda, was a frequent life saver on those many occasions when I would sleep straight through and she would bring my daughter home. Krystal would get very upset whenever I was not able to pick her up, later explaining that it was due to her fear of something happening to me. My little seven year old, going through second grade, was carrying such a burden on her shoulders. It was not long before I learned that many people were not to understand the pressure, the fear, the anxiety this imposed upon her life. Seven years old is a time for care-free playing and learning lessons about the little train that "could". Instead my daughter was learning about cancer, fear of dying, pain and anguish.

Two weeks after returning home, Krystal's second grade teacher called to tell me she heard I was home from the hospital and that she was concerned about Krystal. She said she felt she had given her plenty of leeway while I was in the hospital, but now 'it was time for her to get in line with the program'. My heart shuddered immediately at her matter-of-fact approach to this crisis we were facing, but I tried to hold back my tears and asked to meet with her. My husband had explained the serious issues we were facing but perhaps it wasn't clear. We went to see her again to explain. To explain how life at our house had been far from normal for many weeks now, to explain that Krystal was scared and terrified of losing her mother, to explain that she had not slept in her own bed for over a month, that a different person had been there to pick her up each day, and send her off each morning.

We asked her to help us help Krystal get through this family crisis but we were met with resistance to accommodating the needs of our daughter. It became infuriating to see the blankness on her face and the anguish in ours. When we enlisted the help of the principal we found some relief and Krystal was enrolled in a community program which provides counseling sessions at the school for children experiencing stressful situations.

Krystal's life was vastly improved through this marvelous community out-reach program. Barbara Sachs, a social worker from the Resolve program was truly a God-send for me and Krystal. To obtain this kind of personal assistance was so invaluable in surviving those difficult days when it seemed that no one truly understood what we were going through. I now realize that unless you have 'been there', you really cannot understand fully. I have also come to learn that compassion is not a quality dispensed equally to all humans.

We found later, through further professional therapy, that Krystal was in post traumatic shock and suffering from fear and anxiety. It was so important for her to have an objective party to confide in. She was mature and intelligent for seven years old and did not want to burden me or Warren with her concerns. If she only knew how precious she is to us, that her fears were not a burden. It took two years of therapy to work our way through the many issues that would arise as we all were sent "Navigating Through a Strange Land", a fitting title for another invaluable book I recommend, edited by fellow survivor, Tricia Roloff. This was truly uncharted territory and it was essential to talk about our feelings. Fortunately, Warren and I have always communicated well with each other and with Krystal. We were not afraid to tell each other how we felt.

When Krystal was born I had instituted a practice many working moms may recognize. Since I went back to work when she was only six weeks old, I was determined to have quality time with my daughter. So every night after work, we would take time on our TLC couch (Tender Loving Care) to talk, or sing, or just cuddle. At seven years old, this became our sanctuary. It was a "safe" place where you were free to say whatever you were feeling. Warren and I often used it for our own discussions. This communication is not born overnight but it is never too late to make time to communicate with those important to you. I think too many of us go through life never telling our friends, our families, or ourselves, how we really feel, what we really think, until it is too late or nearly too late.

We are often afraid to hug our loved ones and tell them we love them, maybe due to embarrassment, perhaps our upbringing, or a lifetime of conditioning. I am not advocating syrupy drippy mush, but a dose of TLC now and then can lift the spirit, theirs and yours, and with a brain tumor, why would anyone wait? The worst that could happen is you might be around to tell them over and over and over ...

When God Closes a Door

Having had a total of 35 sessions over a seven week period, I felt the need for a break, taking a month off after radiation treatments finished. Of course, this was contrary to professional opinion that I should act immediately but I needed time not only to recover some physical strength, but also to gather up my senses for a rigorous course of toxic drugs. I needed the time to prepare myself, physically, mentally, and emotionally for something I did not yet understand. It was during this time period that two windows were opened. I was always fond of the saying from the Sound of Music, "Whenever God closes a door, He opens a window."

My youngest sister, Jodi, was really responsible for at least getting the window "unlocked". Twelve years ago I was living alone in New Jersey. Jodi was seventeen and came to visit me and never left. Being her older sister, I felt a responsibility to take care of her for those years before she literally married the guy next door. Now in her own unique fashion, and Jodi is quite unique, she felt a sense of responsibility to care for me. My baby sister has always traveled to the "beat of a different drum" and has the temperament of an artistic creative mind. She had for many years, been utilizing herbal and holistic therapies, many of which I thought were ludicrous. She strongly encouraged me to find a good herbalist or nutritionist to improve my health and as life would have it, voilá, a window flew open.

Through references from many friends, I called and interviewed a number of health-oriented practitioners. Eventually, I found Marcy. I will be indebted forever to my herbal wonder woman. Marcy is a petite woman with the strength and dynamics of an Olympic athlete. Both being of Greek descent, we hit it off immediately. Marcy has studied herbal, holistic, and homeopathic alternatives for many years. She is an intelligent woman whose knowledge of the body and the mind is matched by her compassion and dedication to helping others. She is also a "No Nonsense" type of person which suited me just fine. She says, 'If you are not serious about this, or not convinced, then the alternative approach will not work.'

We began with a very simple approach to using herbs. The body uses herbs, vitamins and supplements to cleanse, burn or build. Different needs are met by different treatments. Since I did not have any background or knowledge in the area, Marcy introduced ideas, information and treatments gradually. While still on radiation treatment, I began by taking only three supplements in addition to my anti-oxidant vitamins: 1) Whole Leaf Aloe-vera juice which I used to calm my stomach and cleanse my system, 2) Acidophilus/Bifidophilus capsules which keep a balance in the bacteria in the intestines allowing the body to better absorb natural nutrients and 3) Liquid Chlorophyll which I learned contained nearly identical components as human blood, (hemoglobin) and cleanses and rebuilds the bloodstream. All this made sense to me considering that Decadron which I was still taking can irritate the stomach and often Zantac or Tums are recommended. With Aloe Vera Juice, however, I eventually stopped needing the Zantac which can inhibit the body's absorption of valuable nutrients. The Acidophilus kept a balance internally, and it is my belief that the Chlorophyll helped to keep my blood counts strong and healthy throughout my treatments.

Marcy also encouraged such mundane 'common-sense but who does it' things such as drinking 64-100 ounces of pure water daily, deep concentrated breathing, chewing food intensely, healthy food devoid of processing wherever possible. Eventually, I would become comfortable with the effect these had on my system and add many other beneficial complements to my program. Over the years since my diagnosis, we have changed my overall program to meet specific needs as they arose. I would soon learn of the benefits of this non-traditional road as I approached my decisions for chemotherapy.

After discussing these alternatives with the oncologist, I was met with the typical response, "Well, it certainly won't hurt you ..." while leaving a long pause that I interpreted as 'but I really don't think they will help.'

While I did not easily find encouragement from the medical profession in general regarding my intention to use alternative natural treatments in addition to my medical program, I did sense there is a "new" attitude emerging on the horizon regarding the use of natural alternatives in medicine. After learning that most drugs were originally plants or other natural substances, but in order to sell them for a profit, they must be synthesized into a chemical product, I lost my fear of trying the natural approach first. I never rule out traditional medicine, because as the baseball player said 'it has been very good to me'. I look forward to a time in the healing world where the two elements will come together and work to truly complement each other.

As one might suspect, I read many of Depak Chopra's books regarding mind and body connection, Bill Moyers' book on "Healing and the Mind", Bernie Siegel's series of books, and many others too numerous to mention.

One simple little book, the first I was to receive came from my sister, Cindy. It was titled 50 Essential Thing to Do When the Doctor Says IT'S CANCER by Greg Anderson, Founder of Cancer Conquerors. At first glance, I thought it was too simple to be of any use in fighting this mighty monster, but it set me up with the right tools from day one. Remembering that David slew the mighty giant Goliath with nothing more than a rock and a sling-shot, I reasoned, why not me?! You see, David had faith that it could be done and later a descendant of David said, 'if you had the faith of a mustard seed, you could move mountains.' So, why not me? Lord knows I had my share of mountains ahead.

One of the simple yet invaluable tools I used, was to keep records of everything and to maintain all of my own medical records. I now have a library full of files of laboratory results, MRI reports along with actual MRIs, copies of EKG's, blood test results, as well as detailed notebooks for each year since my 1993 diagnosis regarding recommendations, discussions with MD's, and follow-up plans. If you cannot do this for yourself due to limitations from a brain tumor, ask someone else to help. If nothing else, get copies of your blood work results; it saves having repeat blood tests done unnecessarily, thereby conserving your personal resources.

Many people grew up in an era when medical technology was rapidly advancing and held great promise to cure mankind's illnesses. Most of us were in awe of the medical profession and its technology. Far be it from us to question, to disagree, to dare to hold our own opinion. We grew up with a respect for the marvels of medicine, forgetting as one doctor put it, "M.D. does not stand for medical deity". Fortunately, the younger generations are far more inclined to want a partnership as opposed to a medical dictatorship. We prefer to work in conjunction with our medical technicians on a fair and equal basis, respecting each other's position. It is your legal right to obtain your medical records and you need not apologize for requesting copies. If you need to pay for copies, it is well worth it in the long run and if it can save your life, just how much would you pay?

Before I checked out of the hospital after my surgery, I put in a formal request for the following:

Hospital Report and Summary
Surgical Report
Copies of Lab Reports and Lab Results
Discharge Report
Copies of MRIs, X-Rays, Pathology Reports

> (Pathology slides are kept by the Hospital but are loaned out for consultation to other doctors, for a minimal fee.)

The hospital medical records department had no problem with my request as long as I had no problem paying the $57.00 for copy time. It was $57.00 well spent when it came time to get second and third opinions on my case. Now, granted, it may be overkill to request all the information I insist on having, but my point should not be missed. It is your right to obtain your records, you are entitled to the information.

Another suggestion from the book led me to the second window that opened for me. Mr. Anderson recommends searching out survivors to find out what they did, their attitude, and draw inspiration from these. So immediately, I began calling everywhere to find someone who had survived a Glioblastoma. I was put on a waiting list for over six months because none of the Brain Tumor Organizations I contacted had any Glioblastoma Multiforme (GBM) survivors I could talk to. This was prior to access to the Internet where now you can find a list of over 1,000 participating people dealing with brain tumors and surviving all types of tumors and all forms of treatment. The numbers for a Glioblastoma are still minimal but if lacking in quantity, we certainly compensate with quality!

When I initially began my search I was down-heartened due to a lack of resources. As it happened, one day after completing radiation, I stopped in at my family practice, just to say "Hi" and let my family doctor know how I was doing. While there, her partner said he had a patient who had a brain tumor several years prior and would I like to speak with her. I nearly leaped over the counter to thank him.

Marla called me that evening and asked what she could do to help. We talked in general and then arranged to meet for breakfast in a local diner. I will never forget that meeting as long as I live. I was so excited, I arrived ahead of time. I had two cups of coffee waiting to meet this real person who had faced what I was facing. Actually, Marla's tumor was an Astrocytoma which was inoperable at the time. Since both tumors contain glioma cells with astrocyte (star-like) characteristics and generally similar patterns, it was close enough in my opinion.

Right on time, in walked this young, beautiful, healthy woman with almost a leap in her step. She had dark brown, thick hair that rested just above her shoulders. She dressed impeccably. She radiated health and I happily found out later she never even had radiation! We recognized each other instantly and dove into conversation as if we had known each other all our lives.

Marla lives in the next town over from me as one of life's many coincidences would have it. We were presently close in age. She told me she was twenty-five years old when she was diagnosed with a brain tumor. She was told the typical 'get your affairs in order', and have a nice life as there was 'nothing they could do'. That being unacceptable to her father, he sent her medical records to every center in the country searching for 'something'. She was accepted into a clinical trial using a combination of three chemotherapeutic agents. She was one of seven who went through the trial. She was one of two who survived.

She was told she would never have children, but informed me that her 5 year old twins defied that prediction. When I found out that her tumor completely dissolved and she has been fine for over 15 years (that was three years ago and she is still fine) I was anxious to know the protocol she followed.

She told me she used BCNU, Procarbazine, and Vincristine and would fly to Buffalo, New York every six weeks to have her dose of whatever, puke all the way home on the plane, and go back to work after each treatment. Aside from being thrilled to know what she had taken and the obvious positive results, I wanted to know if there was anything 'special' that she felt made the difference. I already knew that this was the treatment I would request. I also already knew this treatment had less than hoped for success. More oncologists were leaning towards more aggressive chemotherapeutic drugs. It was sad to realize that in 15 years so little had changed since BCNU or its counter-part, CCNU were still the standard chemotherapy agents used for treating brain tumors.

That day Marla gave me a gift I know I can never repay except to do as she did for me and share it with others. She put it so succinctly, "Rebecca, I had the right mind-set!" I had never considered that term before with the impact that struck me that day. The right mind-set.

Some might call it attitude and Marla and I would probably both agree, we are ladies with an attitude. We are also survivors - long term survivors. All the long term survivors I have met regardless of the disease seem to have a common thread. A very dear friend recently commented on this phenomenon. He noted that while he had searched out every possible treatment, every new therapy, and left no stone unturned in his search to help his dear friend survive, he noticed that the people who survived all seemed to have a certain resolve, a conviction within themselves that they were survivors. It was not the therapy or treatment as they all took different paths, but there was a commonality in a strong attitude. Marla had that strong, positive, determined attitude and eighteen years later, she is here to tell about it.

It suddenly became clear. As one gentleman said, "You have to make a conscious effort to live. You have to work at living, take care of yourself, eat right, sleep right, and you need to have a purpose." I wasn't clear on my purpose yet, but that was not the critical point at that time. It was knowing that I had a purpose in being alive.

The right mind-set has to do with the way you look at the positives and negatives and the part you allow them to play in your life. The right mind-set has to do with attitude. It is positively positive about achieving the best possible outcome. It is determination to determine your own destination. I speak redundantly because there is no second guessing yourself when you have set your mind to something. I set out to create my own mind-set before reaching the next hurdle in my journey.

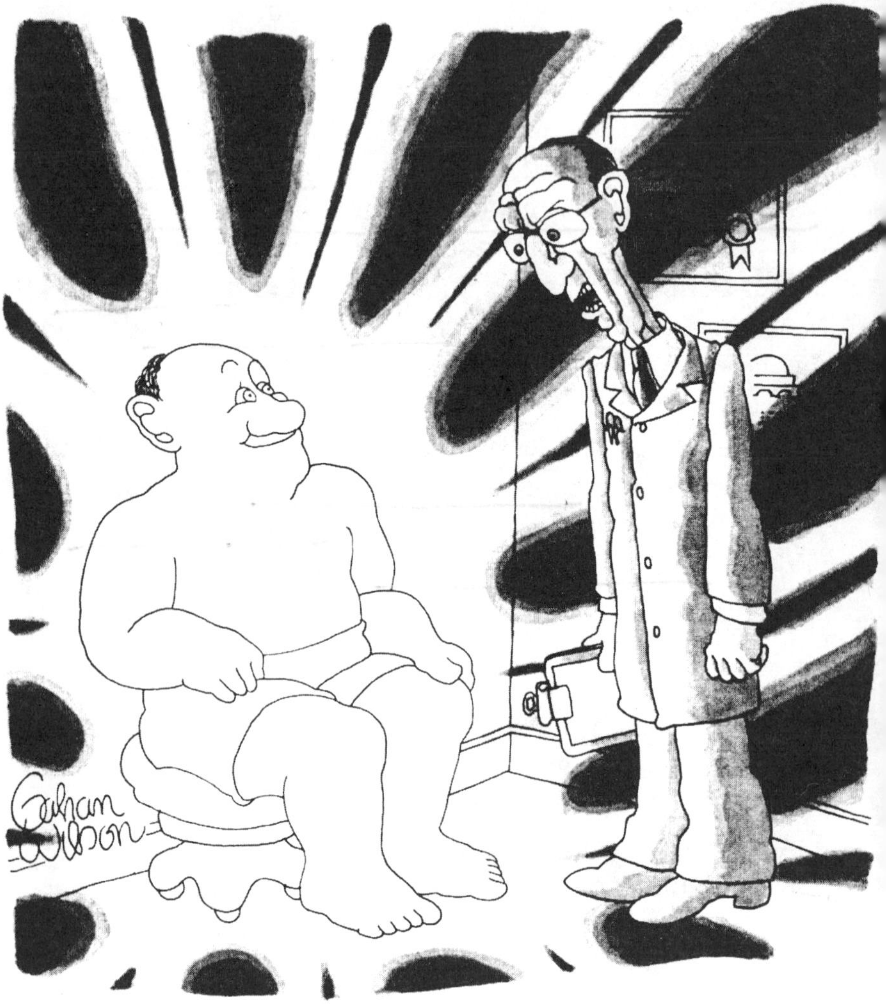

"You've been fooling around with alternative medicines, haven't you?"

Chemo Cares
Chemotherapy Treatment

With bated breath I waited to hear the results, after a month post radiation therapy. My MRI (Magnetic Resonance Imaging) scan showed no "remarkable" change which in my case was a good thing. It always bugged me when doctors said something good was "unremarkable". I thought that since there was no sign of tumor, it was "VERY remarkable." I wanted to leap for joy. I wanted to celebrate. Remarkable, indeed. With no visible tumor, the peripheral rim of the tumor site had been radiated effectively. Except for lingering tiredness, I felt fine.

After having decided to decline the high dose chemotherapy with stem cell rescue, I met with my oncologist to discuss a plan of action. I was sitting in one of the examination rooms on the only available seating, the examination table. I felt uncomfortable, not physically but psychologically. Dr. Lowenthal came in with his brisk and cheery manner all intact. He seemed a bit too cheerful for the occupation he practiced but I gave him an "A" for effort. I suppose he was trying to make me feel comfortable, but I felt at a total disadvantage sitting there like a sick "duck" on the table while he stood looking down at me. Although it may have been quite unintentional, from this angle he was forced to talk down to me. The net effect was that I felt he WAS talking down to me. I wondered if doctors were aware of the impressions they give their patients. I wondered if patients ever mentioned their discomforts half as often as I was inclined. After all, here is someone who is "suppose to heal you" of cancer, you better not get him upset with you.

Nevertheless, it occurred to me later to request all future consultations be conducted in the doctor's office. After nearly twenty years in the insurance and financial industry, I had many doctors come to my office to discuss their financial health. I offered them a seat in a pleasant office and made every effort to make them comfortable. I felt entitled to the same professional courtesy. Of course, if an examination was necessary then the examination room is appropriate, but for consultation and discussion of treatment, I maintain strong feelings about using the office. I prefer to be treated with respect, face-to-face, when discussing which alternatives are available and be in a position to ask the necessary questions.

I have been met by some silent and not so silent resistance from nurses who are following standard office procedures, from doctors whose offices are too cluttered to utilize, and others who are just confused that they never thought of it, but more often than not, it has worked to my satisfaction. I once voiced my feelings to a very high profile neuro-oncologist. Without the slightest hesitation, he jumped up on the table and sat next to me, much to my amazement. His associate interns and my husband sat bewildered in the chairs below. It was wonderful to have my feelings validated by his positive reaction. Thank you, Dr. Hochberg.

After advising Dr. Lowenthal about my decision not to proceed with the more aggressive chemo, I explained my per chance encounter with Marla and hence my decision to use the same chemotherapy protocol that she had used; BCNU, Vincristine, and Procarbazine. That is, if he didn't have any objections. I realize now, in looking back on the situation, that I was determining my own treatment plan. Some people might call me assertive, some may consider me aggressive, and others might consider me down right obnoxious. When they walk a few moons in my moccasins, then they may judge.

Dr. Lowenthal was gracious however, and agreed that it made sense to try this approach. I would begin with an infusion of BCNU on Monday. Warren accompanied me to the oncology office where there was a room set up with comfortable recliner arm-chairs. Most of the chairs face a long "picture-window" with a view of the trees behind the office. I picked my seating as I was the first person in at that early hour: a recliner in front of a sunny window to look out at the bird feeder attached to the outside.

I love to watch birds, as I often do from my kitchen windows. The striking red cardinals nest in the tree above the garage and hop from fence to fence looking for food for their youngin's. There is sometimes a hummingbird in the morning glories, and once a woodpecker knocked his way into my heart and maple tree. However, in the eleven months of going back and forth to Dr. Lowenthal's office, I never recall seeing one bird at the feeder. I think they knew they were too close for comfort to toxic substances and kept a safe distance. I felt that if I could have had the option, I would have done the same, but since I had chosen to include this medical modality in my program for survival, I decided to make the most of it.

BCNU and CCNU are long standing chemotherapy drugs used to treat brain neoplasms (tumors). They are both derived from Carmustine. Zofran, a recent medical marvel, is an anti-emetic to minimize the side effect of vomiting. My new oncology nurse, Nancy, sat in her laboratory mixing up this chemical cocktail as I settled into my seat. She was pleasant and as patient and kind as the day was long. And that day was long. The BCNU burned, the drip had to be diluted with saline so my veins could tolerate it and it took over five hours to infuse into my tired veins.

After the BCNU infusion was completed, I would return in a week to get an intramuscular injection of Vincristine. I would remain at home while I took Procarbazine, the third chemotherapeutic agent in my program. This drug came in pill form and was taken two or three times a day for two weeks. At the end of the Procarbazine fest, I would return to get a final injection of Vincristine. During the next four weeks I was allowed to recover from the four weeks of treatment, and the process would start over again. Thus, became the cycle of Four On and Four Off. Ultimately I would receive a total of six such treatments spanning an eleven month duration.

Warren watched painfully as Nancy hooked up the IV drip, stuck my vein and adjusted the flow. It took several adjustments and several dilutions with saline solution to get a mix my veins could tolerate. The clock on the wall ticked away the minutes slowly. We chatted to take my mind off the burning in my veins but after a while there was little left to talk about. It was more painful for me to watch Warren watch me so I decided that although I was grateful for his presence on this initial trip, the rest of the time I would manage on my own.

Unlike radiation, although my spirit was willing, my body was not up to the commute. I was not able to drive myself with great confidence after the arduous treatment so to ease Warren's mind, we arranged for drop off and pick up from the 'Chemo-Plant'. Warren, along with many friends and family pitched in their services and re-arranged their schedules to be there to pick me up or collect Krystal from school if I was late. Once again, my network of dear family and generous friends, did not fail me. I actually had more volunteers than I needed. It is a blessing to have such friendships in life and I had many when I needed them.

Just as it was time to begin on my first Procarbazine regimen, my parents came to stay and help with the many things that were piling up while I went through the chemotherapy. Bills I usually took care of were accumulating, Krystal needed help with school and homework, the dog was not getting her usual walks as I had slowed down from radiation and needed to conserve energy and strength. Things were beginning to take their toll as I am inclined to be organized and my house now felt upside-down. I was grateful for Mom and Dad's arrival and the respite it offered.

Having taken the Procarbazine pills early that morning, just as we sat down to dinner I ran upstairs and began wretchedly vomiting. It was so violent, I could not stop even when there was nothing left to heave. I hung my head over the bowl, its coolness seemed to bring some relief, although hugging a toilet is hardly my idea of relief. Warren stayed by me the entire time, rubbing my shoulders, giving me water to rinse my mouth and a cool wash cloth to wipe my face. As soon as I took the slightest sip of water, the heaving started all over again. This went on for hours, until I finally insisted Warren call the doctor. "I don't care if it is the middle of the night - I can't go on like this," I sobbed.

Most people tolerate Procarbazine better, but for some unexplainable reason I have a propensity to be that 1-in-a-million girl, always seeming to fall within the narrow 1 percent corridor of life. Ha, I really don't believe that. Every time I talk to another brain tumor survivor, we compare notes and find we have the same or similar symptoms and have been told the same or similar anecdote, "We've never had anyone experience this before." Does anyone really keep track of who is experiencing what? Does anyone really know the affects these drugs can have on an individual human body - during treatment (early stage), post treatment (2-6 months) and late onset (2 years ad infinitum)?

Following one unusual medical symptom, I was referred to the neuro-surgeon who said it wasn't from surgery and sent me to the radiologist who said it wasn't from radiation and sent me to the oncologist who said it wasn't from chemotherapy who sent back to the neuro-surgeon. When I complained about going around in circles and getting nowhere, someone blamed it on my 'hypochondria'.

I have come to view this allocation to the one percentile corridor as a blessing in disguise. If I really am that one-in-a-million, then I can be the one-in-a-million to survive!

Dr. Lowenthal and Dr. Malkin both recommended using an anti-emetic to manage the drug, Procarbazine. Compazine was recommended as the first line of defense since Zofran costs an arm and a leg. Unfortunately, Compazine did nothing to ease the nausea and the big guns of Zofran were called in to finish the job. At the doctors office, I took a liquid form of Zofran before the BCNU; at home I took Zofran in pill form prior to my dose of Procarbazine. With the Zofran, the nausea resolved itself. Even with the relief of the new drug Zofran, we both could see this wasn't going to be easy. At the end of two weeks taking Procarbazine, it was time to return to the oncologist's office for a final shot of Vincristine. After a four week break to recover from this regimen, this four week course was to be repeated five more times. I couldn't imagine how I was going to endure it.

The chemotherapy was clearly something I had to psych myself up for. Often, when the day was over and we would settle down for the evening and Warren would lean over to kiss me goodnight, he would find me with tears in my eyes, a lump in my throat, and fear in my heart. I sobbed so often on his shoulder, telling him how scared I was. I am not ashamed to be afraid nor of the tears it brought on - it is one of the most real and penetrating feelings I have ever known. I have been mugged, robbed, assaulted and threatened at gun-point. I have been on a small plane in a lightning storm. I have been lost alone at midnight in Harlem. I have had both feet broken at the same time. I have had a ruptured appendix with blood poisoning, and now most recently, an emergency craniotomy for a malignant brain tumor. I've even experienced natural child-birth. I think it is fair to say I have known pain and have been intimately acquainted with fear. However, I never knew this fear.

I never knew the fear that accompanies lying awake at night wondering whether there would be a tomorrow to wake up to in the morning. At the conclusion of a busy day, just when you should be relaxing into a refreshing nights' sleep, this nocturnal fear creeps up and ties a knot around your throat. It won't let go. You cannot will it away. You cannot laugh it away or make it disappear like the daylight sometimes allows. Night fear has a stronger power. Your thoughts unwind and crawl out of the corners of your mind whether you want it or not. They slither down your neck and chill your spine. They wrap around your being, suffocating your will. Nothing is as clear as you want it to be. The 'what if's, the 'but's and maybe's take the place of 'surely and of course'. My daily resolve dissolves leaving me in a heap of terror and dark shadows.

Warren takes hold of my shoulders and hugs me tight. His strong voice is filled with resolve and determination; the determination I cannot find within myself. He gives it back to me. He insists everything is going to be fine, and although I do not always believe it, I always love to hear it. His strength is imparted to me. I draw on his courage and know I cannot disappoint him. It is unacceptable to him and to me to let each other down, especially in this fight.

Fear is a paralyzing emotion and can inhibit your ability to think straight, take action, even to think through your options. But fear is a useless emotion unless it motivates you to do something positive. I have always found that in order to rid myself of some unpleasant thought or feeling, it was necessary to replace it or edge it out, with something uplifting, positive, cheerful. So I found it to be with fear. Replace it with anger, with mirth, with resolve. Push it back, way back, and soon it loses its power over your mind, over your body, and over your will.

Somewhere along this fascinating but terrifying journey, I came to a fork in the road. There were two signs, one to the right pointed to Happiness, the other to the left pointed towards Misery. Of course, I am speaking metaphorically, but for everything in life you have at least two choices. Every choice, it must be remembered, bears consequences. I knew I had only two choices in dealing with my cancer: I could choose to search out happiness in each day, or I could allow myself (another form of choice) to be miserable over my misfortune.

This is an opportunity in life to find out what you are made of. Yes, you may need to pull yourself up by your bootstraps occasionally or you can sit there and be "down" all day. Yes, you can feel sorry for yourself, no one should have to deal with brain cancer, or cancer of any kind but life is full of injustices - the victory lies in how we conquer the injustice. It is your choice.

My friend Diane tells the story of how she was left high and dry by her dead-beat husband when her son was just an infant. She looked at her baby, and said, "Well honey, we can sink or we can swim, but Mommy is a swimmer and that's what we are gonna do!" She came out on top as did her son - stronger and more compassionate.

Now some oncologists may cringe at what I am about to share, but I decided that every visit for my chemo-therapy treatment was going to be a picnic -- literally. Since conceptually, chemo is no picnic, I decided to make it one otherwise. I packed a delicious, healthy lunch, all light food, nothing odoriferous, a piece of fruit, a few crackers, pure water. I brought a good book and my cassette player with head phones. I arrived with a good cup of coffee in the morning - yes, I still have to have my caffeine, sorry folks.

After Nancy hooked me up to the IV, I settled in with a blanket, pillow and heating pad, pushed the chair back and relaxed listening to my favorite music. Later I would have lunch, followed by planned exercise around the office. Yup, Dr. Lowenthal's office was set up with all the examination rooms and doctor's offices on the outside walls. In the center was the laboratory. This left a lovely square corridor to do my daily walking.

Exercise has always been an important part of my life, but as my life was being threatened from more things than one, exercise was one of the few things I could still do for my well-being. It gave me that much needed sense of control and although I was hardly training for the New York marathon, I was indeed training for the marathon of my life. With the IV pole, bag of saline, bag of BCNU, headphones and cassette playing, I would walk around the square for a half hour, 15 minutes one way, 15 minutes the other. I often wonder whether he or his partners ever were aware of my routine. As they would see me wandering one way and then the other, they probably assumed I was lost. I was - lost in my own thoughts about getting well.

I am sure that it would be chaos if everyone did this at the oncologist's office so I am not promoting it on a grand scale, but it would be nice if it were possible. After my exercise, I would take a nap. Then I would read or talk with other patients. I noted the anxiety and strain of many who were there. I knew that if someone could talk to them about other things, it might help them forget, at least for a time, why they were there.

One day, I was relating to another cancer patient about my ordeal with relentless itchy skin. I was telling her how I searched high and low trying one expensive treatment after the other to ease the itching to no avail until I was told about a very inexpensive cream called, "Oh, what was it, Tri... something." The gentleman sitting next to me straightened up and blurted it out correctly saying to me, "Are you talking about Triamcinolone?" "Yes, how did you know?" I asked, immediately recognizing the correct name. "Because I am the chemical engineer who invented it some twenty five years ago," he said with a bit of pride in his voice, and he added, "good stuff, huh!" "Great stuff", I answered, "I could just kiss you for it!" He blushed modestly but was obviously pleased. It made my day a bit brighter and I'll bet it did the same for him. Life is uncanny - if you open yourself up to the wonderful possibilities, you never know who you will meet along the way.

On another eventful day, I had to use the bathroom so I scuttled myself with gear and tubes into the lavatory facility. As I was getting my self put back together, I accidentally pulled the IV tube out and liquid saline began to spout everywhere. I called for help but no one heard me from inside the bathroom. Since I could only use one hand, I could not reattach the tubing that was now wildly flinging itself all over spilling its contents. Finally able to get to the door, I called for help and Nancy came rushing in to save me from total embarrassment. I always said, "What I wouldn't do for a dull moment!"

My chemotherapy began in March of 1994. At the end of the first month, Warren decided I needed a vacation and reward for getting through the tough treatment, knowing it was a long rocky road ahead. We all needed a change of scenery so Warren came home one day with tickets to the Island of Nevis.

I had never heard of this tiny resort hidden in the islands of the U.S. West Indies but what an unexpected delight. It was a long plane trip with a stop in Puerto Rico and a short jaunt to St. Kitts, one of the larger islands. A very dear friend of ours had moved to St. Kitts a year earlier. Rhea and her husband Jeff picked us up at the airport in St. Kitts. We had to take a boat ride to the secluded island of Nevis. Rhea and Jeff are working on new condominiums which are being built on the island of St.

Kitts. We toured them all, wishing we could stay longer. The following is what I wrote in my diary about our very special trip:

> <u>March 28 to April 1, 1994</u>
>
> We left on Monday and although it was a long trip getting to this island paradise, it was well worth every minute. I loved it and I love Warren for taking me there. It was so relaxing, fun, beautiful and romantic. We had breakfast every day on the veranda over-looking the ocean, surrounded by red hibiscus. We talked and enjoyed being together.
>
> Krystal got her hair corn-rowed with colored beads and was ecstatic! She loved the pool and stayed in all day. I love the way the hotel staff catered to our every whim. They came by the pool daily and spritzed you with cool water and handed out cool face cloths. Talk about pampered!
>
> Rhea and Jeff came over and Warrren and Jeff got a game of golf in while Rhea and I relaxed over lunch by the pool. We went to their place on our way home on Friday, high on a mountain with three fabulous windows facing the blue-green ocean. Rhea gave us a tour of the island to show us the monkeys and the spectacular views as she explained that St. Kitts has numerous monkeys inhabiting the island. Unfortunately we never saw a one, until we reached this tiny hidden cove on the far side of the island. We had Mango Coladas at a little bar on the beach and Krystal fed the tame monkey that hung out at the bar. I'll go back again, I hope.

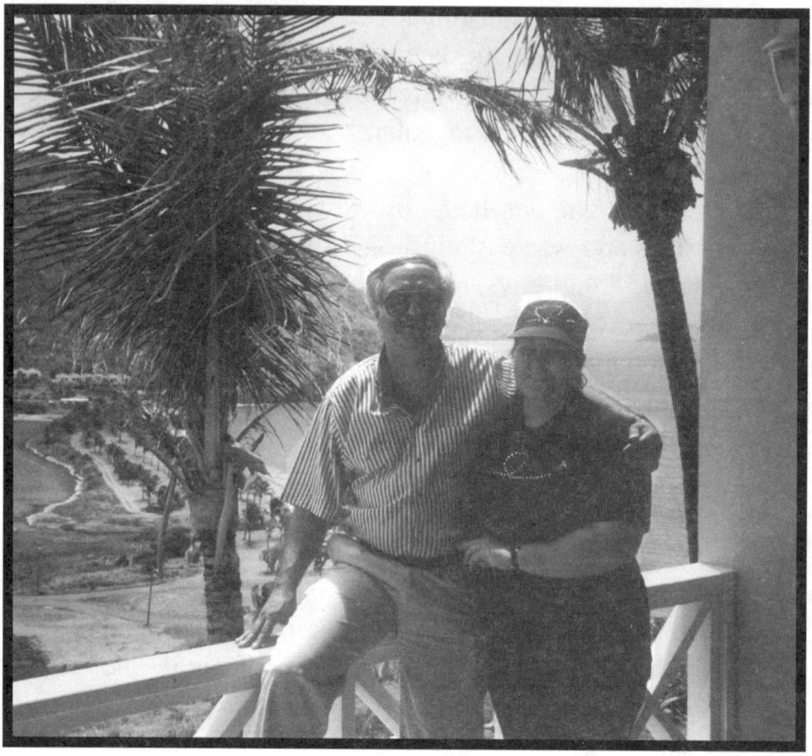

Warren and the Pillsbury Dough Girl
in Paradise

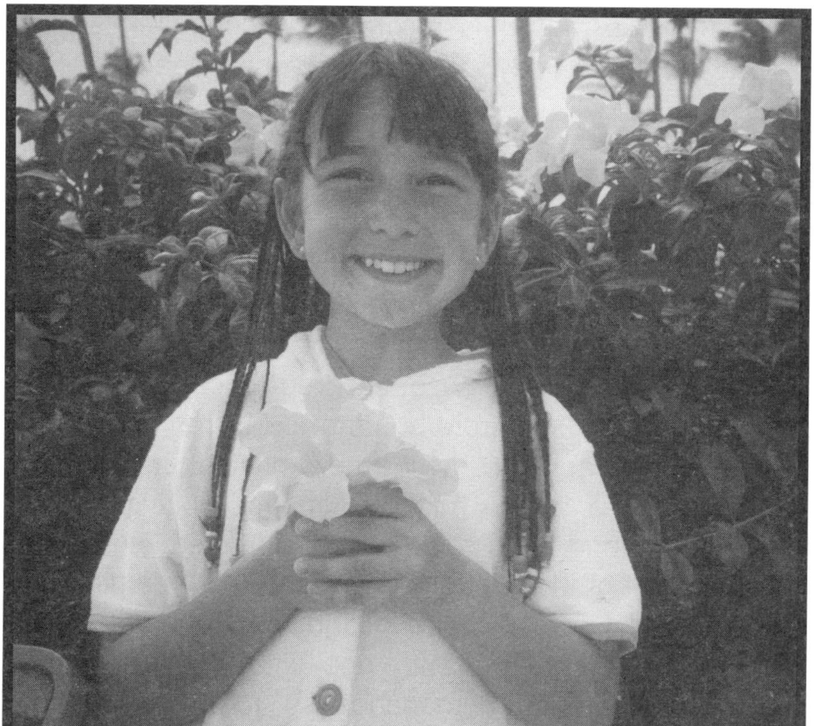

Krystal in Nevis
With Corn-Row Hair

Ten months into my treatment my resistance was wearing thin. Most people have trouble maintaining their White Blood Cell (WBC) counts during the harsh regimen. Thanks to my herbalist, however, I had been taking liquid chlorophyll for several months now. Not once during the eleven months of chemotherapy did my White Blood Count (WBC) fall below acceptable levels, although it did decrease from my pre-chemo levels. I believe it was the liquid chlorophyll's components that help to boost the body's ability to replenish healthy blood cells.

Nevertheless, I am no super-woman, and I was tired of taking these drugs. I also intuitively determined that my body had taken all that it could withstand. It was around this time that I began to notice little red spots on my skin which were beginning to itch with increased intensity. Within a few days, I was covered once again with incredible huge welts from head to toe. The "itch witch" had returned and this time the anti-itch cream that worked so well before had little impact. My skin was burning. My endless scratching made matters worse but truly was out of my control. I was literally scratching my skin off and I was in burning agony. Benadryl which usually knocks me out with one little pill was barely making a difference in megadoses. I was not getting much needed sleep as the itching kept me awake throughout the night.

My complaints seemed to be met with skepticism that any of this had anything to do with the chemotherapy. It was determined that the Procarbazine had not induced the rash and I had not yet had the final phase of Vincristine. Ultimately, it was determined that I had developed an allergic reaction to the Zofran, once again putting me in that lonely 1% category. Since I only had one more treatment to go, I requested a cease fire to the program. I figured it had surely done all the good it was going to do by now, so why prolong this agony?!

Dr. Lowenthal and others, however, knew the potency of the tumor we were attacking and strongly recommended that I continue the full program to its conclusion. Against my own reservations, I agreed to the final session. Due to my allergic reaction to Zofran, I was switched to the newer anti-emetic, Kytril which worked quite effectively. As a new drug at that time, it was only available in liquid form for intravenous infusion. It was nearing the holiday season when doctors become unavailable and I wanted to end the year with an end to the Chemotherapy. I was hoping for a clean slate heading into 1995.

Dr. Lowenthal's oncology nurse was scheduled for a much needed vacation the same time that my last treatment was to begin and Dr. Lowenthal was also going to be away. Since I was really opposed to carrying over treatment into January, it was suggested that I have the treatments done at home by a visiting nurse. My long-time friend, Lois, who is a paramedic, introduced me to an excellent home health-care nurse. She came and set up my chemotherapy drugs but due to the distance told me she could not administer them and that she would teach me how to do it.

I freaked. Just simple hysteria, nothing more. Me, inject myself? I don't think so.

In a panic, I called Lois and at 9:00 p.m. she rushed over to my house to help Warren and me figure out how to administer the drugs. It was suppose to be simple, but my veins were so burned out from all the stabs and scars, they had basically collapsed from over-use or abuse. Even Lois with her years of experience had trouble getting the line into the closed and unwilling veins.

In an effort to get a suitable position, Lois had to climb up on my bed to reach a usable vein. She was so kind and gentle and finally found a vein in my hand that she could use. The port was left in my hand for the next infusion and Lois or the visiting nurse returned to change it periodically. The veins were so small, the infusion was slow and painful and sometimes it wouldn't even drip at all unless Warren held the bag at a certain level. There I lay on my king-size four-poster bed, pathetically hooked up to an IV that my husband had to hold up over my head to utilize the laws of gravity.

When Lois said she would teach Warren how to do the infusions in the future, Warren looked like he would faint - his usual dark complexion faded to a pale shade of gray. His warm loving face froze at the thought of needles and tubing and the pain it was causing me. I smiled as I told him this was his chance to get even for all the misery I caused him over the years.

The poor guy had jet black hair before he met me, now it was quickly turning a distinguished silver. I grinned and told him I had confidence in his hidden medical talent. Warren is a mechanical engineer by education, and an environmental engineer by profession so I knew he could handle a little needle and some toxic drugs.

In just a few days, he was snapping those hypodermic needles and setting up IV lines like an experienced medical professional. I teasingly called him Nurse Warina, a pretty daring thing to do while someone is wielding a needle in your face!

At the end of the Procarbazine treatment my body told me loud and clear what I already knew - ENOUGH ALREADY! I was weak and tired but not so tired that I could not keep the following diary:

> *12/8/94*
>
> *Met with doctor Lowenthal and all the rest of his patients this morning where we discussed cutting the Vincristine to 1/2 portion and using a nursing service to administer the IV Kytril. Also discussed my cessation of menstruation for the entire room to hear. Remind me to thank him for sharing this with complete strangers.*
>
> *12/15/94*
>
> *Had shot of Vincristine and 2 Procarbazine shots after Kytril.*
>
> *12/16/94*
>
> *Asked for stronger pain killer. Denied. Nursing service asked. Denied. My friend, Sharon called doctor's office at 4:45pm and Nancy said*

O.K. Started on 2-3 Percocet. Thank you, Sharon.

12/16/94 pm

Nurse couldn't get catheter in arm - did IV into right hand - O.K.

12/19/94

Krystal came home sick. I began to have pain in abdomen. Pain was intense and unrelenting. Asked Krystal to get help, I was doubled over in pain. She called 911 and police called an ambulance. Rushed to ER with Krystal in ambulance holding my hand. She called her Dad at work and told him to meet us at the hospital. They wouldn't let her stay with me so she sat alone in waiting room, waiting for Warren to arrive.

I was examined by ER doctor who said nothing was wrong and left me laying there from 1pm until 4pm. Doctor on call examined me and said I had a severely impacted colon. He reached up to my neck (not via my throat) to 'break' the obstruction. Also gave me injection through my IV without checking or sterilizing - it burned.

12/19/94 pm

Lois checked and found needle in catheter was bent as I suspected. Removed from right, put in left hand. Hurts a little but O.K.

12/20/94

Feeling better but will lay low. Called Nancy about last treatment. Waiting call back.

12/20/94 9:30pm

Nancy advised no more chemo - Vincristine caused impacted constipation - cannot take a chance again.

12/22/94

Dad came to visit - left this morning. Had major allergic reaction by 7pm. Red as a lobster from head to toe. Nurse requested OK to give Epinephrin - near anaphylactic shock - later went on Decadron and Benadryl.

12/27/94

Going through Decadron withdrawal again ...

1994 Summarized

Allergic Reaction to PCB (Procarbazine)

Allergic Reaction to VIN (Vincristine)

Allergic Reaction to Zofran - switched to Kytril

Impacted Colon - rushed to ER

Catheter for Home IV would not work

Used outside IV on hand - got infected

Finished with chemo

Missed last few days of PCB & last shot of VIN

OK with me!

1994 is O V E R !!!

Thank you, G O D !

Who's on First?

In the course of chemotherapy treatment, I felt the need to expand my comfort level with the path I had taken. I felt it was right based on the knowledge I had, but I did not feel I had all the knowledge I needed. It was early summer when my sister-in-law told me about a doctor her father had seen at Massachusetts General in Boston, Massachusetts. She had inquired about whether he knew anyone in the neuro-oncology field in Boston and he referred me to Dr. Fred Hochberg.

Without thinking to ask anyone's permission, I called saying I had been referred by Dr. "XYZ", I had a Glioblastoma and I would like an appointment with Dr. Hochberg. A third pathology was done and an appointment was arranged.

Since I had retained copies of all my scans and medical records, I Federal Expressed everything to Dr. Hochberg's office prior to my appointment. Warren and I drove to New Hampshire to leave Krystal with my Mom and Dad, and then drove into Boston to meet with Fred Hochberg, M.D., a neuro-oncologist and Associate Professor at Harvard Medical University.

There we were met by a delightful young lady from Ireland. Bernie was so helpful and ushered us into an examining room. Dr. Hochberg had reviewed my scans as well as a pathology report done by Massachusetts General Hospital. He would be in after his interns did an overall review.

It was the first time I had actually had an extensive neurological evaluation. They tested my reflexes, my walking capacity, my balance, depth perception, as well as sensitivity to touch, slight pain, left and right brain functions. Again, it seemed they were impressed by a lack of any physical or cognitive deficits from the tumor or the surgery.

When Dr. Hochberg came in, I was awe-struck by the rugged good looks that placed him in the movie-star league. But looks and demeanor aside, I was totally impressed with his expertise and knowledge as well as the comfort he made me feel during our conversation.

He was complimentary of the results of my surgery, which I told him were due to Dr. Beyerl's expert hand. No doubt sensing I had consulted with a number of experts, one of the interns asked the appropriate question, "Who do you intend to have in charge of making decisions about your treatment?"

I know it is professional courtesy not to interfere with the recommendations of another professional, but I did not understand the politics of medicine. My doctors in New Jersey were aware I had sought a second opinion at Memorial Sloan-Kettering but they had no idea I was meeting with doctors in Massachusetts. It seemed to me that I had every right to meet with whomever I wanted without anyone's permission. I never meant it as discourteous - this was my life and I was merely attempting to save it from being destroyed by a Glioblastoma Multiforme Grade IV malignant brain tumor. The more professional opinions and medical information, the better my chances of succeeding, I thought to myself.

In answer to the question posed regarding who was in charge, I simply said, "I am." The young intern looked surprised so I continued politely, "Let's make it clear right up front. I am here to get the right information, medical advice, and a qualified professional evaluation of my options, but make no mistake, I make my own life decisions. Not my husband, not my parents, not even my doctors. So if you are asking who's on first, the answer is me! I respect the knowledge you have and it is my hope that you are willing to be consultants to my situation."

Dr. Hochberg seemed to understand immediately that I was there for his expertise, professional opinion and his advice, but not his assuming responsibility for my case.

He indicated that my tumor site was nearly imperceptible on the MRI scan. I was elated to hear this for the first time. He said I was doing, "Remarkable", and I sensed he didn't get to say that as often as he would like. Apparently the treatments were working but further evaluation using additional technology might give us a more complete picture.

Dr. Hochberg recommended a PET scan (positron emission tomography) which takes clearer pictures using heat sensitive dyes that highlight the areas of the brain where there is active cell growth. The scans indicate in color areas where a tumor is actively growing, if there is necrosis (dead cells), and can provide more depth of information regarding the tumor site.

In addition, he recommended a CBV or Cerebral Blood Volume scan also called a "Fast MRI". The Fast MRI takes pictures at a much faster rate, thereby showing more definition of tumor. We arranged to have these additional scans done as I was deeply interested in what these they might reveal.

As the incredible professional he is, Dr. Hochberg dictated a detailed letter to my doctor in New Jersey including his recommendations and evaluation. He suggested I have a DLCO or Diffused Lung Capacity evaluation since BCNU causes lung fibrosis. I was nearly five months into treatment and never had my lung capacity been checked or even mentioned. When the test was done, I discovered I had lost 40% lung capacity. No wonder walking the dog had become such a chore.

Instead of wasting time pointing fingers, I headed straight for my herbalist practitioner to see what we could do to correct or minimize any further damage. Marcy gave me an herbal combination of Marshmallow and Fenugreek and some herbal teas.

Within days of taking these natural expectorants, I was expelling whatever was in my lungs causing impairment. Fortunately for me, I took it upon myself to seek a third and valuable opinion or I might have had permanent lung damage from the BCNU. Over the ensuing months, my lung capacity was restored to normal as I continued with the herbal alternatives.

Over the many months of treatment, I had much opportunity to think about this matter. It became clear to me that I had to assume the responsibility of healing and helping myself and that every medical professional was there to assist in the process.

It was my job to ask the questions, get the answers, make the decisions. It was their job to provide the medical expertise, make medical recommendations, and support my decisions. I had the choice to abdicate all power to my physicians but then I had little part in the outcome. No, my choice was to make my own life decisions and never regret the outcome.

Dr. Beyerl and Dr. Lowenthal were somewhat surprised when I excitedly told them I went to Massachusetts General Hospital for further evaluation and the resulting recommendations. In that illuminating 20/20 hind sight I realized, then, the need to be sensitive to your doctor's feelings as well as your own.

This is a learning process for us all and in my enthusiasm to survive the role I had been assigned, I may have stepped on a few toes and made a few politically incorrect assumptions. My formal apologies to anyone I may have offended.

The medical profession needs to recognize this type of assertion not as a threat or an insult but for what it really is - a desperate need to leave no stone unturned in making an intelligent decision, especially when it means your life. After talking with Dr. Beyerl about my need for a third opinion, I asked him, "If it were your wife, what would you have done?" He smiled graciously and said, "I get your point."

The PMS Syndrome
(Pre-MRI Stress Syndrome)

For most of us in the world of brain tumors, Magnetic Resonance Imaging scans, called MRI scans, become a way of life and you become accustomed to the routine. A typical routine for me goes as follows:

1) I arrange them early in the morning because my patience level is high and my stress level is low.

2) Pre-arrange to get copies to bring to the doctor's office. It is a colossal waste of time to show up at the doctor's office and find the scans have not. And relying on the written report is futile.

3) I also coordinate them with an appointment with the doctor for either the same day or as soon as possible. There is enough anxiety about the scan without having to wait days for the results.

4) Sign in and answer the questionnaire. No metal parts allowed, inside or out. That

means pace makers, metal devices, as well as jewelry, hair pieces, etc. CT (computerized tomography) can be utilized if you happen not to qualify for the MRI scan.

5) The typical MRI machine encloses most or all of the body in a long tubular cylinder which is open on both ends. It is imperative to lie perfectly still while the imaging pictures of the brain are being taken. I lie on my back on the conveyor; it is cold and hard. It curves up slightly and the nurse straps me in and I mentally prepare to enter this tiny 'tunnel of love'. I call it that because usually the tunnel is so snug you end up hugging yourself for the entire hour. I happen to be claustrophobic. Since I have trouble in elevators and crowded grocery stores, it became imperative to devise a method to deal effectively with the MRI.

6) To deal with the claustrophobia, I bring along my favorite CD and most MRI technicians are very agreeable to playing music other than the choices offered at the MRI center. I bring, of course, my favorite Jimmy Buffet CD's, but also, the Three Tenors, Harry Belafonte, Frank Sinatra, The Phantom of the Opera, and even Patsy Cline have accompanied me through my MRI's.

7) I usually need a blanket as the room is generally a bit too cool for comfort. The technician hands me a bulb-like squeegee-thing to squeeze if I need any assistance during the MRI. They will also periodically ask if you are OK and you can answer. However, because of my fear of being "enclosed" in anything tighter than my blanket, I close my eyes before I go inside the machine and DO NOT, I repeat, **DO NOT** open them until the entire procedure is complete, including the in and out time for the dye injection.

8) Once inside you will hear your music until they begin the actual scanning which sounds akin to a jack-hammer blasting through concrete on the streets of New York City. It drowns out the sounds of Pasty's crooning "Crazy" but she's already singing in my mind, so I can take it from there.

9) In order to see the tumor or tumor site more distinctly, doctors often request a scan be done with contrast dye as well as without. The dye is injected intravenously so the scan stops while they search out a usable vein. After three years of being poked and prodded, my veins are not the least cooperative and it now takes some extensive patience (not one of my better qualities) to get this portion completed. The dye feels cool as it makes its way up my

vein and past the brain blood barrier into the waiting host, my wonderful brain.

10) During this procedure of approximately one hour, I relax to the sounds of my music, my breathing, and focus in on deep relaxation techniques. I tell my brain everything is OK (sometimes I believe it and sometimes I don't). I visualize warm comfortable colors that imply health, i.e. light purple and warm greens. I made the mistake of telling the technician at one scan that I see an array of warm and serene colors before they inject the dye, and after the dye they become very cool soothing blue tones. He looked at me cross-eyed and walked away shaking his head. I walked away wondering if he had ever even been inside the machine he operates daily.

After a year of scans every three months, I began to notice a pattern of extreme anxiety just prior to having an MRI and an intensified level of anxiety trying to wait patiently for the results. I would get so crazy because sometimes the doctor's office would set them up just before he was going out of town and I would be left going out of my mind.

Assertiveness training told me that I would have to resolve this unacceptable procedure. I explained to the Office Manager that I had what is called PMS, PRE MRI SYNDROME and that my symptoms were extreme anxiety and relentless stress if required to wait long periods of time to find out the results of the scans. She was extremely sympathetic to me and now does everything in her power to arrange the MRI and my doctor visit as close together as possible. We have formed a great partnership and her assistance is something I could not do without.

After one scan, she knew the doctor was away but she obtained permission to call me and let me know the written report indicated the results were fine. It made waiting for my appointment with Dr. Beyerl the following week a lot less stressful - I even looked forward to sharing the good results with him. After all, my success is his success too!

For one particular scan, I had gotten so crazy that I asked the doctor to check them while he was at the hospital and just tell me if it was OK prior to my appointment. Dr. Beyerl, my neuro-surgeon, has been so considerate and aware of the effect these scans have on me and he has graciously accommodated me when possible.

For the first two years after my diagnosis, scans were done every three months to monitor closely any possible signs of recurrence or regrowth. This type of tumor, glioblastoma multiforme, is the most aggressive form of brain cancer or brain tumor. There are microscopic cells which cannot be seen but which, if activated, can double themselves every twenty-one days. One can imagine at that rate it would not take long for a recurring tumor to occupy a major portion of the brain, threatening life with each new cell.

In fact, it was recently discussed at a brain tumor conference, that it takes a million cells to even be visible on an MRI scan, so at that point, you are dealing with a lot of cells out of control. In fitting paradox, it was noted that the best time to treat a tumor is when it cannot yet be seen. Of course, using current technology, this is nearly impossible. However, with research and funding, the future may hold some long overdue technology to make earlier brain tumor detection, diagnosis, and treatments to prevent rampant growth.

Being well aware of the nature of these tumors, Dr. Beyerl is cautious about keeping ahead of the beast and sees me on a regular follow-up basis. After three years, I was having trouble getting an MRI done every three months. As I explained to my physician, "You have the month before the scan to worry, the month you have the scan and get the results, and a month to de-stress yourself, before it is time to repeat the whole process again. I just can't handle it being 'so in my face' all the time."

Thankfully, Dr. Beyerl agreed to order a scan every six months as opposed to every three months as of January, 1997. He feels that I have become very aware of anything that may indicate something is wrong and I will call if I feel it is necessary to check sooner. However, often I have some obscure symptom which has required us to err on the side of caution rather than taking a cavalier approach.

The Impatient Patient

Ask my life-long friend Robin what my worst quality is and without a doubt she will say my impatience. Ask my daughter how I drove before the tumor and she will tell you 'very impatiently'. When she was three and seated in the back seat of my car, we approached a traffic circle where we slowed down. A deep little voice from behind me impatiently said, "Com'on, buddy, MOVE IT!". Obviously she heard that somewhere before, I am NOT proud to say. The proverbial apple fell so close to that tree it hit me right on the head!

I willingly admit that patience was never one of my virtues. I despise lines at the movies, lines at the grocery store, lines on the highway. I get uptight having to wait in 'waiting rooms'. Even pregnancy made me impatient - for nine and a half long months!

Therefore, it is fair to say that my current impatience as a 'patient' has deeply entrenched roots. Now, however, I get impatient for totally different reasons. No longer stuck in the working mother 'rat race', I drive like an old lady and it is the people behind me who are beeping their horns. Going mid-day to the grocery store is virtually line-free and as for movies and shopping, I am just happy to be alive to complain about the lines.

My impatience now comes in the form of intolerance. I have little patience for insurance companies who make you wait for endless reviews just to qualify for an MRI scan.

I get impatient with the endless amount of paper work required to 1) see a competent doctor, 2) obtain the proper treatment and 3) get a claim submitted and paid. With all this paper work, my doctors' offices now have five to seven non-medical staff personnel.

I have little tolerance for the new "referral" system now in use by many managed care insurers. This was suppose to cut cost, be more efficient, and deliver better service. Whoever sold that bill of goods could sell ice in Alaska and we would pay for it. I am now required to see a doctor I don't need to see, to be referred to a doctor I do need to see. Call me silly, but now I have paid for two doctors when I only needed one. Where is the savings in that?

I also have no patience for the new fangled telephone answering systems in use by most companies and services, including doctor's offices. If you want this, press that, but if you want that, press this, followed by the 'pound' key, followed by 'all of our representatives are busy, please hold ...'. I have no patience for holding. If you were told you had only months to live, would you want to spend any of it 'HOLDING?!'

I have no patience for Government Offices that maintain long lists of telephone numbers and short lists of people to answer questions. Again, a person could grow old just waiting to get through or, worse yet, they might get permanently lost in the maze of telephone options. If you are fortunate enough to reach an actual "live" person on the other end, either it is their first day and they know nothing or it is their umpteenth and they will tell you nothing.

I have no patience for hospitals that make you re-register information into their computer every time you go for out-patient services. Isn't that why you have computers, so once it is in there, we don't have to repeat it again? Or do we need to justify the five ladies doing all this data entry? I might have patience for it if the same hospital had not cut its nursing staff so they cannot find a competent person to locate a vein. I say keep the nurses and skip the registration.

I have no patience for nurses who have no patience. One nurse recently told me after ineffectively stabbing me several times, that "my veins didn't like me and were hiding." I looked her straight in the eye and said, "It's you with the needle, they don't like."

Well so much for my 60-second Andy Rooney imitation regarding my impatience with the world. I am trying hard to be a kinder, gentler person despite the obvious character flaw.

I would like to share some helpful information on a few useful subjects you may face after being diagnosed with a brain tumor.

Health Insurance

By the time you are diagnosed with a brain tumor, you are pretty much stuck with the insurance you have, so hope for the best, but by all means make the best of it. Check your benefits before any procedure and do not hesitate to call the claims office first to check coverage for a particular procedure as well as the reasonable and customary cost covered by your carrier. It is advisable to make copies of all your records.

Do not be afraid to appeal a denied claim. If you can medically justify your claim to a "higher authority", often the initial decline can be overturned. If it is a life-saving treatment that has been declined as experimental, consider legal assistance as well as the assistance of your medical professionals. A letter from a medical professional to the Medical Director at the insurance company can go a long way towards resolving your inquiry. Go up the insurance corporate ladder until you are satisfied. Unfortunate but true, it is the squeaky wheel that gets the oil.

Organize your health records. I keep a file of all the lab reports, a file for all MRI written reports, and a file for insurance company claims for each year since my diagnosis. When medical records are needed they are readily available. You may need records for your tax accounting, or for a new physician, or to check a treatment or medication that worked, or one that caused a reaction. A medical diary has been especially useful after brain surgery when short term memory is in short supply.

Disability

Most states provide some sort of short term disability benefit for which you apply through a state agency. Some companies also provide short term disability through formal or informal salary continuation programs. After short term disability (STD) benefits are exhausted, you can apply for Social Security Disability benefits as well as corporate sponsored Long Term Disability benefits. Some provide a benefit to age 60 or 65, others for a specific duration (2 years, 5 years, etc.). While the definition of an eligible disability is strict for Social Security approval, many brain tumor survivors qualify. If you qualify by Social Security standards, chances are you will qualify with any corporate plan.

Long Term Disability (LTD) benefits - most plans coordinate with Social Security for a maximum benefit limit.

It appears many people are embarrassed by the idea of filing for a disability claim, as if it were taking advantage of the system or indicated a personal failure on their part. While I strongly agree no one should abuse any of the benefits available to them, remember you paid for such protection over many years of work the same way most pay the premium for their health insurance. Utilizing benefits you elected to purchase may help you recover from your condition so you may return to a productive life. Many are intimidated by the process. However, it can be simplified using some of the following suggestions:

1) Ask the Social Security Office for everything they will need in order to process your claim for disability benefits. Make a list and be sure to have the correct forms as well as dates, signatures, and notarization if needed. Be sure to retain copies for your personal records.

2) Obtain all the needed information, including copies of doctor's statements. Do not allow them to be sent separately to the Social Security office. They will likely end up lost and cause untold delay. Once you obtain all required information, send a cover letter briefly explaining your disability and a list of the forms being submitted. Be sure to include Social Security numbers, Employer statements, dates of birth,etc.

3) Try to get the name of the person who will handle your application and, if possible, their direct extension or the dreaded "voice-mail".

Social Security offices are filled with over-worked and under-paid personnel who appreciate someone who makes their job easier by providing everything they need to make a fair evaluation.

It is worth noting that after two years on Social Security Disability you automatically become eligible for Medicare coverage.

Wills, Life Insurance, Living Will

You may have been told to "get your affairs in order". As one Glioblastoma survivor said, "Everyone should have their affairs in order." Sadly, that just isn't so. My feeling is, if I get everything in order, I'll never need it so that is reason enough to do it. If you don't have one, get a legal will immediately. If you die without a will, you are in essence leaving your decisions and choices up to the courts in the state in which you live. Do you want them to decide what happens to your family and your assets? If you do have a valid will, have it reviewed; laws have changed and many people are not aware of the terms of their will.

Investigate and decide on a living will. A living will is different from a regular will in that it is specifically designed to address the issues regarding life support. Here you can relieve a heavy burden placed upon family members about whether to maintain life support if you become mentally or physically incapable of making your own choices. Make sure your Executor/Executrix has Durable Power of Attorney should you become disabled and rendered unable to sign legal documents.

In addition to a legal and up-to-date will, you may want to consider writing a letter of intent to be included with your will. If there are personal items, memorabilia, or sentimental things you want to have passed on to someone specifically, and it is not stated in your will, you may want a letter of intention signed and dated by you. This will serve to clarify anything you intended to be passed on to a specific friend or family member. It states things like I want this ring to be given to my sister, (sister's name) or I want my favorite rocking chair to be left to my grand-daughter (grand-daughter's name). It is not necessarily legally binding, but it does state items promised to loved ones specifically and leaves no question as to your intentions. A great deal of irreparable damage has been done to many families fighting over such matters.

Life Insurance

Review your life insurance benefits, riders, and options. You may have the right to increases without providing medical evidence of insurability. You may have Waiver of Premium benefit which means premiums are waived in the event of your disability (after a specified Waiting Period). You may have Disability Income benefits as a rider on your life insurance. Be sure your Executor/Executrix knows about the policies and their Policy Numbers, has access to them, and knows where to call for information. Review your beneficiary and ownership arrangements and update if necessary.

Check with the Employee Benefits Coordinator at your company for company provided Group Life Insurance, Group Short and Long Term Disability Benefits, and Group health policies as well as the conversion privileges available should you leave employment. Also inquire about your company's policy on COBRA continuation or current laws in effect regarding continuing your health insurance should you be terminated from employment (especially if the termination is due to disability).

Review Individual Disability Income contracts which may have increasing benefits and Cost of Living adjustments while disabled. Typically, the premiums are waived during disability.

Check out any Long Term Care benefits to which you may be eligible. This is a relatively new benefit which helps to cover costs of Home Health Care not covered by medical policies. It can provide benefits for at home care or in nursing home care. Some larger corporations may provide such benefits as optional. These benefits usually follow a waiting period and are for a limited duration.

Financials

Be sure your trustees are aware of all the bank accounts, savings and checking accounts, safety deposit boxes, safes, and investment accounts as well as identification codes or keys needed to access the information. Make sure your beneficiary or Executor/Executrix is aware of 401K plans and provisions as well as IRA's and pension plans, etc. List all credit cards and card numbers and amount of outstanding debts.

Of course, for some stricken with a brain tumor, many of the above items will have to be taken care of by a family member or trusted friend. When you are caught in the throes of crisis, it is easy to get overwhelmed. Do not be afraid to ask for help. Ignoring these difficult issues will not make them go away and will only make the task harder on loved ones.

Maintain accurate receipts of your out-of-pocket medical expenses for your accountant as you may be eligible for a medical deduction on your tax returns.

The point is to take care of what needs to be taken care of so you do not have the stress lingering from uncertainties. Do the best you can and then put the worries away with the paperwork. I could not say it better so I'll let my fellow brain tumor survivor, Marylou sum it up, "Everyone out there attached to mother earth should have their affairs in order out of respect for 18-wheelers!"

Coloring Outside the Lines

Curled up in my favorite corner of the living room sofa, I was often found reading two or three books at one time. Somewhere in all my readings, I came across a phrase which captured my attention as well as my imagination. It simply read, "Only a few who got well, did so without coloring outside the lines." It reminded me fondly of something a former boss used to say in reference to my ability to get things done, "you are not afraid to go outside the lines to achieve your goal." Now as I look back, I see that my whole life has been an experience outside the 'lines'.

I remember as a child growing up in New Hampshire with my brother and two sisters as well as my seven cousins who lived right next door. We would all get new coloring books and crayons and see who could do the best coloring. It seemed that everyone else could color inside those big, black lines; everyone except me. Not surprisingly, I liked going outside the lines and enjoyed creating new colors by coloring over one color with another. I liked coloring the background putting in my own sky, clouds and sun, or green grass in the areas most kids usually leave blank. At forty-two years old, I recently sat down to color in a large coloring book my sister sent (for my daughter, of course). Even now I could see the same tendency to want to color beyond the boundaries, make my own definitions, to personalize my picture. It was childish fun and it was delightful.

Coloring outside the lines means pushing beyond the pre-determined limitations. In order to get well, you must be willing to risk pushing some boundaries. You must be willing to go beyond what is known, documented, proven. You need to define your own palette, filled with the colors you want in your life. If you have to color over a color, no problem. Perhaps you will end up with a totally different color all together, or a totally different dimension in your life. Perhaps the colors will be richer, deeper, enhanced with passion and bring a deeper meaning to your life. Perhaps by searching within and without, you will transform your life from a faded water-color to a bold, bright Picasso; a warm and tender, Renoir; a daring and colorful, O'Keefe.

This artistic metaphor may be too esoteric so I will explain exactly how I colored outside the lines, pushing boundaries I had not known before the brain tumor. One way was to tip-toe softly into the world of alternatives, herbal medicines, holistic and homeopathic healing, just testing the waters enough to be sure it was safe. With all the medications doled out by medical practitioners, I proceeded with great caution, checking to see if there would be any interference or interaction with my traditional medicines and the new herbal alternatives. I admit to being skeptical in the beginning but the more I personally investigated the more I was convinced these alternatives were indeed improving the quality of my life.

Moderation is my recommendation for medicine, traditional and non-traditional. Having been asked literally by hundreds of people, how much did I take of this or that, I must honestly say, it is different for everyone, different at different stages of treatment and survival, and even differs at certain times of the year, the weather, and my specific objectives. There is no pat answer, no black lines, so to speak. You must define your own comfort zone.

Although taking pills is something I truly hate, today I have over forty different holistic, herbal, or homeopathic alternatives I choose from daily. I still take my "pediatric" doses. That's just me and it feels right. It has been suggested that the dosages I use are not strong enough to affect a flea but I can live outside that line.

I read about a study conducted where people were given a medication for a duration of time. After the treatment was completed, they were given a pill that looked identical to the one they had been taking, however, it was a placebo, and they were informed that it was such. When doctors checked these patients after using the placebo, they found that the body had continued to produce the same chemicals as the former medication produced even with the placebo. This was an incredible demonstration to me that the body can be coaxed into doing some remarkable things.

It is truly amazing that we have put men on the moon, yet we know so little about the mind/body connection. Even with all our libraries of books and medical journals, our medical professionals, researchers, as well as scientists, we have barely tapped the surface of what we need to know about this incredible human computer. Did you know that the brain weighs less than 3 pounds yet a computer capable of handling a single brain's output would cover the entire earth? The brain sorts one hundred million (100,000,000) bits of data ... each second, yet uses far less electricity than an average light bulb... - *Mainliner Magazine*, March 1978 pp 43-44. Pretty incredible.

In addition to the basic anti-oxidant vitamins, I took a 'super' vitamin C which contains seven different variations of Vitamin C. I also immediately began use of Shark Cartilage and Essiac Tea. I read Dr. I. William Lane's book, Sharks Don't Get Cancer and called him directly on the telephone to discuss this treatment. I decided using Shark Cartilage supplements "wouldn't hurt". Essiac Tea was originally a remedy used by Native American Indians. As the story passed on to me indicated, it was given to a nurse whose name was René Caisse, "Essiac" being her name spelled backwards. She began to notice many of her cancer patients improving after using the tea. She brought her findings to the National Health Institute and some notable cancer centers but, bureaucracy being what it is, there were never any scientific studies conducted. My reasoning was, do I want to wait for the NIH or any other organization to draw the lines for me? Coloring outside the lines is habit forming.

In addition to the herbal medicine, I searched for other alternatives to healing. I reasoned that I needed to exercise my brain the same way I needed to exercise my body. I have always subscribed to the adage, 'when the mind is tired, exercise the body; when the body is tired, exercise the mind'. It appeals to a sense of balance. Now with the monstrous threat being made to my mind, my memory, my right and left brain coordination skills, and my very thought process, I felt compelled to do something to truly exercise my mind - to stretch it's capabilities, develop deeper grooves, to strengthen its capacity.

At thirty-eight years old, I had never played a musical instrument, had no musical talent or experience except for playing the radio and a pure enjoyment of all varieties of music ranging from The Three Tenors to Billy Ray Cyrus. My only exposure to piano was taking my daughter to her weekly piano lessons.

Sitting there waiting for her one afternoon, it dawned on me - THIS was the perfect mental and physical exercise of the brain. I could not think of another non-strenuous exercise that included the coordination of the left and right hands, left and right feet, fingers playing together, singularly, up the keyboard, down the keyboard, in different directions simultaneously, eyes reading a completely new foreign language, memory and brain harmoniously joined in this complex effort to create the ultimate reward: beautiful music. It was the perfect therapy - for me.

If you had the good fortune to have learned to play the piano as a child, thank your parents for the great gift. As an adult, it can be the most frustrating, embarrassing, arduous task, severely testing the mental powers of endurance. I will never again take for granted the simplest of melodies after struggling to pound them out

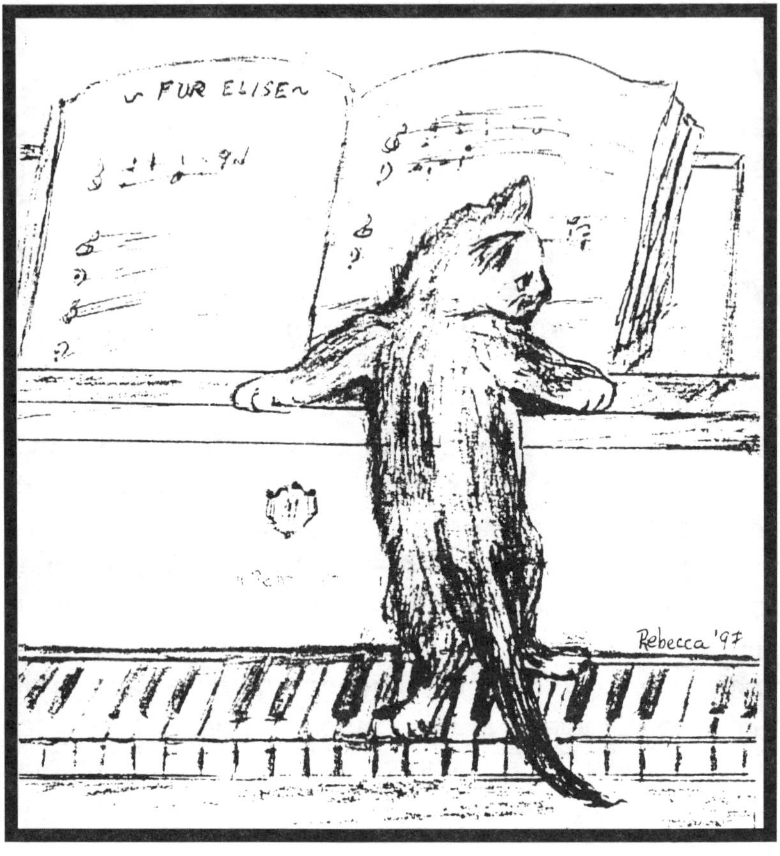

Für Elise
Our kitten, Demi, on my baby grand

on my "baby grand". Often the frustration of feeling like a fool and a failure has left me hunched over the keyboard in tears - but not once have I considered quitting. My two piano teachers have both been compassionate people who despite my obvious lack of natural ability, not to mention my limitations, have been gracious and supportive of my efforts. They have understood this effort for the therapeutic benefit it offers. They have encouraged my weak attempts and applauded my courage. They have inspired me to higher expectations for my own abilities and capabilities.

What I lack in talent, I hope to make up for in appreciation for this rewarding endeavor. However, if I never learn another song, I will feel satisfaction in the knowledge that permanently etched into my memory board are the notes to play "Ode to Joy" from Beethoven's Ninth Symphony as well as Beethoven's "Für Elise". Not bad for an old lady with a brain tumor!

After adding the piano to my repertoire for healing, I embarked on another path leading me to many new modalities. I explored the wonders of massage therapy, reflexology, yoga exercise as well as meditation, visualization and, of course, prayer.

Esther was my first massage therapist but when she moved to Israel, she introduced me to Abby who has become not only my massage therapist but also a valued friend. The quality of my life has been enhanced by her skillful therapy as well as her knowledge of the body. The chemotherapy treatments wreaked havoc on me and I continue to feel the after-shocks even now. My body was not capable of recovering from the treatments on its own. Massage therapy has helped to set it back on course. It has served to de-stress the muscles, tendons, and ligaments damaged by three years of significant inactivity and toxic treatments. It has helped my body in healing and strengthening itself. It also provides a haven of tranquility and peaceful relaxation.

It is Friday, the end of a long achy week. I arrive at Abby's looking forward to the therapy session. She checks my chart and asks what is concerning me this week. I get comfortable on the massage table, covered with sheets and warm flannel blankets. Abby turns on the music. Melodic sounds of nature fill the room: gentle water falling, birds softly chirping, harmonizing with the background sound of a flute. The scent of almond oil with a gentle touch of lavender essence is in the air.

The medical massage lasts for an hour. It warms my muscles, kneading out kinks and knots with a tempered ease. I concentrate on my breathing: deeply in, gently out. Stress and anxiety melt away like the scented candle burning nearby. My thoughts are calm. No matter what I walked in with, the cares of the day are lost, rubbed out of my mind, out of my body.

I especially savor the almond oil and lavender essence as the aromatherapy touches all of my senses. With my eyes closed I envision the warmth of the pale violet light, healing my mind and body - leaving me feeling ethereal, light, uplifted. At the conclusion, my mind and body are in a state of complete relaxation. I breathe a final sigh of relief and leave to face my world again.

At the beginning of massage therapy, my body was so battered and bruised internally from the toxins it had been given, I could only endure a very gentle, soothing massage. My muscles had atrophied from a lack of use and would easily be strained. A deep rub was just too painful. After a year of therapy, we have made tremendous progress. Abby is now able to massage my head, my neck, and my muscles without causing any pain. Many of my arthritic symptoms have dissipated and the torn ligaments are beginning to heal.

After chemo, it was so easy to pull a tendon or ligament with a sudden sneeze or a quick movement. I tried chiropractic therapy but truly preferred the medical massage. However, both can stimulate healing and reduce stress. Although previously considered outside the medical boundaries, these therapies are now being accepted as healing aids by many medical professionals making it easier to 'color beyond the traditional lines'.

After attending to my needs, I am in a much better frame of mind and body to attend to the needs of others. My primary concern is my husband and my daughter. Knowing that time is not limitless, I decide to make every moment count. Why put off today the pleasures that will make tomorrow's memories?

Every year since my tumor diagnosis Krystal and I put together a list of projects we will try to accomplish for fun. This effort has led to our building a dollhouse which we painted and decorated to look similar to our own house. We used the same wallpaper we used in our house, same linoleum from our kitchen, and furnished it for Krystal's Penny People dolls.

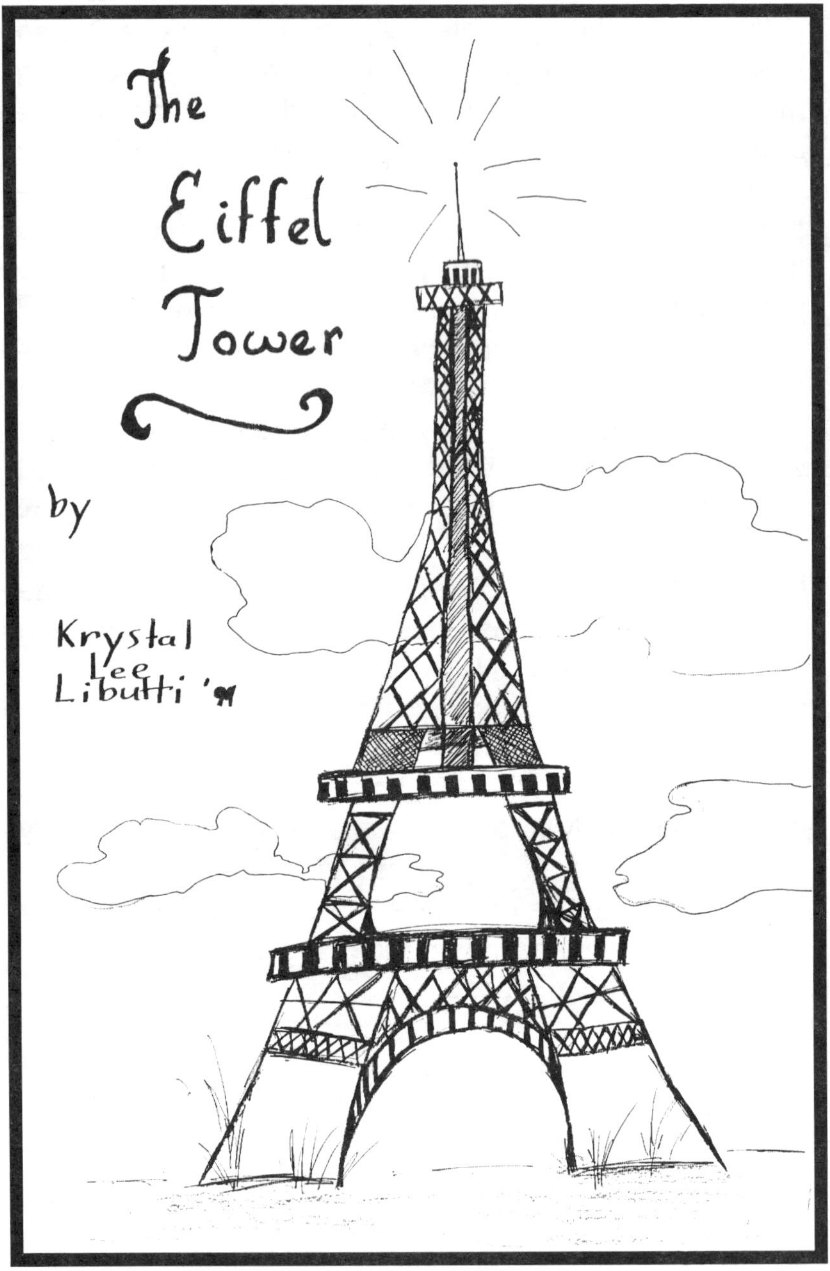

In 1997 We Saw The Real Thing

Another project involved putting together a 3-D puzzle of the Eiffel Tower, a place we both hope to see in person in the near future. We also, with the help of my friend, Virginia, made porcelain-like dolls with eyes and eyelashes, hand-painted faces, hands and feet, and made a beautiful dress with green velvet and lace trim. We styled the doll's wig and tied the long curls in a big ribbon. She now sits proudly with Krystal's other special collectibles. I am confident that this one will hold cherished memories for many years to come.

Since Krystal is a doll collector, when I saw an advertisement in the local newspaper that a well known doll maker was coming to town for a children's benefit, I brought her to the show. We took pictures with Yolanda Bello, the famous doll designer and had her sign the back of her doll to Krystal in person, adding another special memory that will endure a lifetime.

Together during the first spring following my surgery, we planted a number of rose bushes and irises. The following year we were delighted by the abundant roses, each bush carrying a different fragrance and color, as well as a regal bloom of tall and elegant blue and purple irises; the reward for a few back breaking days of planting. With each year's new blooms, I am reminded of the blessing of renewed life and I thank the Creator of such splendor.

Another project was to create an exquisite bird house for the blue birds. I read in the newspaper that the blue bird at one time was abundant in New York and New Jersey but none had been seen for many years. In recent years, a few had been spotted in Long Island, New York.

So Krystal and I put together and hand painted a house for the 'lost blue bird'. It had a painted door, a window-box with painted flowers, and we hung it in a tree outside. By spring we found a tiny nest of twigs lay inside. We don't know if it was a blue bird but it was a safe haven to one of God's tiny creatures throughout the long cold winter.

The therapeutic value of these projects cannot be calculated in dollars and cents. But it glows in the smile of my daughter, the blush in her cheeks, and the sparkle in her eyes when we labor over these projects together. Together we have found so many ways to color outside the lines and together we have healed. Warren has joined our endeavors with his own unique talents. He has spent many hours building Indian houses with Krystal, making a colorful fish aquarium, growing a crystal 'garden', taking her out on the golf course or to the putting range. They go fishing together on every vacation to New Hampshire and its many lakes. We sit out on the jetty and I help with the bait and they fish. Our memories are works of our art, our inspiration, our joy for life and each other and while we keep pictures in a photo album of many of our 'projects', we will hold these moments within ourselves for a lifetime.

Hire, Fire, and Back-Fire

After traveling the medical highway for many miles, I detected a measure of cynicism creeping into my attitude. I am not sure if I am cynical by nature or if it is a fine art I have honed over many years of being naively duped into thinking someone else had all the answers. I suspect it slowly evolved from a dissatisfaction when the answers did not make sense.

It had been suggested to me that modern-day medical professionals were merely 'highly trained mechanics of the body' who could be hired and fired at the will of the patient. It certainly made sense with some of the medical technicians I had encountered and I initially adopted the idea. It was certainly empowering to realize that doctors work for you, and while their services are greatly needed, they are also well paid by most citizens. Some forget that even with a generous health insurance program, it is the patient who has paid the premium over many years to insure the benefits received from the medical field.

While health care is no longer what it used to be, the services for many of the "specialists" come at a very high cost. And if you want the best you usually are required to bear the cost. Since you are ultimately the one who pays for the services, either directly or via an insured health plan, you also have some say in what is done, how it is done, and just who you want to do it. If you are not satisfied with the service, just as with any other profession, you have the right to "fire" one and "hire" another.

This emerging attitude towards the medical profession in general has often been fueled by unpleasant treatment, arrogant professionals, and a threat to some perceived control. But I have learned some very valuable lessons regarding the way one treats medical professionals as well as the way we want to be treated by them.

For the most part, nearly all the medical personnel I have encountered have been warm and compassionate professionals. A few have been a bit aloof, but their technical competency was never in question, hence a cool distance was acceptable. A few, and I still think that is a few too many, were less than professional. I have chosen to share a few examples so others might identify similar encounters and make changes that could possibly save their life. Sometimes, it is that critical.

When I had fully completed my chemotherapy, I decided I needed to know how my immune system was faring after the highly toxic exposure it had received. It seemed logical that if I was going to build up my immune system to fight this cancer I needed to know where I was starting. Systematically, I went down the list of my health care providers requesting a test of my immune system. I was quite well aware that this simple blood test is done on a fairly routine basis for patients suffering with AIDS.

However, after calling over twenty doctors and being turned down for this simple request - some claiming it could not be done, others suggesting it was a waste of time - I was forced to look elsewhere.

Finally encouraged by one doctor to whom I was referred by a colleague, I called and explained my request. He said he could help. I drove to upstate New York which was not an easy task for me but I felt strongly about my mission. After telling my story for an hour while he sat there pondering without a word, he slowly rubbed his beard in a long thoughtful gaze. I thought he was going to respond with some great revelation, when he simply said, "I am not the person to help you. My secretary will give you a referral to Dr. So and So before you leave."

I was stunned into silence and drove home shaking my head and wiping away my tears of frustration. Not long after the incident, I received a bill for $250.00 for his time. In utter disbelief, I responded with a brief but pointed note, "You did not do anything to earn this fee and I will not pay you for wasting my valuable time." I have not received a response to date.

Not being one to surrender, I pursued my quest to find someone who could test the degree to which my immune system may have been compromised by my treatments. I was intent on continuing my use of herbal alternatives to help my immune system, so I continued my search. I was once again referred to a doctor in Pennsylvania who would not only do the test, but fully explain the results. It was encouraging to walk into his office and see his many degrees from places like Johns Hopkins and Memorial Sloan-Kettering.

When the results came back, he called me immediately and had the results faxed to me. He was quite impressed that my immune functions were all within normal range except for the "killer cell count". These were the cells that kill off abnormal cells generated by the body. My "killer cells", he indicated, were double that of a normal healthy person, which we figured was why I was still here to talk about it. No one can say with any certainty how accurate the results are, nor can we pinpoint the reason for such a healthy immune system, but no one can completely rule out the effect my herbal alternatives had on my survival. Whether fact or fantasy, I felt vindicated by the good news.

At approximately the same time, I embarked on a mission to lose the excess weight I had acquired during the phases of treatment. I admit to being a "stress eater" and the previous two to three years had certainly supplied sufficient stress with which to contend. It seemed to me that so many things had been taken away from me by this deadly disease: my health, my energy, my body, my hair, my ability to have children, my career, and above all, my sense of security. I don't smoke and I couldn't drink alcohol, play my favorite sport of tennis, jump and shout in my favorite aerobics. Food was the one last thing that offered such a comfort - the last hurrah! It was a security blanket that eventually I would come to feel was smothering me.

I tried all variations of diets and programs. At Weight Watchers, I was duly encouraged, until week after week, I stayed at the same weight despite adhering to the program. I tried Beyond Pritikin, with much the same results. In the quest to overcome the overwhelming weight, I was once again referred to a 'Biochemical Nutritionist' as he called himself. He required a substantial payment up front and then faxed me a one-page copy of his plan. This exclusive program is known as the 'salmon/salad diet' because you eat mostly fish and vegetables. After fifty-five days on this strict regimen my body finally let go of ten pounds, hardly a tremendous success but a step in the right direction.

However, in the midst of following this highly restrictive program I had questions and concerns which were not being answered by this 'guru' of nutrition. I was getting frustrated, light-headed, and nauseous but I hung in there until I received a call from his secretary telling me that he no longer wished to work with me and would prefer to refund my money. Suddenly the shoe was on the other foot, so to speak. I was on the other end of being fired by the guy I hired to help me!

Initially I was indignant but, after some introspection, I began to see some irony in the lesson. The right to hire or fire can back-fire if you are not careful. It was an amusing lesson until he decided not to refund my money. To add insult to injury, I regained all the weight and then some in record time. I lost money, gained weight, and hurt my pride. Chalk that one up to experience.

After much frustration about my weight, I returned to my family physician, discouraged by my failure and with a number of questions listed on a notepad I always carry to the doctor's office. After explaining my need to lose weight, she in essence told me I should just be glad to be alive and learn to live with the extra weight. I tried to explain how much stress it was putting on me emotionally and physically. My cholesterol was over 400 and I could not function with this much weight. My feet and legs were cramping, my arches were giving in, my back was aching. She looked at her watch and said, "Well, I see you have more questions. Your fifteen minutes are up so you'll have to make another appointment," as she headed for the door.

I made another appointment but I made it clear I would only see her partner and I wanted my records transferred to indicate a change in physician. I do concede this problem of time has been created by managed health care and the constraints it places on doctors. Again, this is where the public domain must voice their dissatisfaction.

There is a medical crisis brewing which is likely to change the nature of medicine as we know it. The doctor/patient relationship needs a bit of overhauling in my opinion. In general, it is up to the public to define the terms they are willing to accept and at what price.

I now not only have a greater and deepened respect for the wonderful professionals I've met along the way, but I also have a greater compassion and understanding for the courageous people on the receiving end of this diagnosis. As tough as any doctor's job may be, a survivor's job far exceeds it. Survivors don't have the advantage of years of medical schooling. They have a crash course in survival within a matter of a few days, weeks or perhaps months. They have no manual to guide them, few precedents to follow, and little time to assimilate data. The role models in the world of brain tumors are few and far between.

While no one can hand you a manual to follow, experience is often the best teacher. It is this experience of brain tumor survivors that must be shared and passed along.

Perhaps a data-base of survivors and their treatments will yield the clues necessary to solve the mysteries of the brain. I applaud the many who are trying and hope for their success.

Most problems in life can be resolved if both sides maintain mutual respect. Doctors have a tremendous and arduous occupation. The majority meet the challenge. That is not to say improvements cannot be made. I now realize that doctors often distance themselves from their patients to maintain a certain objectivity and a measure of self-preservation. However, the doctors who have been most healing to me are those who reached beyond the boundaries of medical protocol and touched upon the simple fact that their patients are human. They may be scared, ailing or frail, but they are not incompetent, nor powerless. Most are simply in need of encouragement, optimism, albeit, cautious optimism, and not least of all, hope to achieve their personal best throughout whatever medical condition has afflicted them.

Hope can only inspire the best possible results. It is in keeping with the foremost objective of the medical ethics, "First, do no harm". Most people look to their doctors as beacons of knowledge, not recognizing that knowledge is not unlimited on every aspect of each medical situation. It is not humanly possible to know everything and doctors, we've discovered, are human. For that reason alone, no doctor can or should make predictions for one's life expectancy. In spite of dismal prognostic statistics, many survivors have surpassed the expectations of their physicians. Perhaps many more would achieve better results with the right encouragement.

One lovely lady comes to mind. Twenty-five years ago she was diagnosed with a Glioblastoma Grade IV brain tumor. There was even less effective treatment at that time and she was told back then that she might 'have a few months'. She outlived the doctor who gave her that prognosis. Within four years, she had a recurrence of tumor and a second doctor gave her the same dismal prospect. He retired before she did. Twenty years later and now a mother of one son, she was evaluated by a third doctor who said it was impossible for her to have had a Glioblastoma - she would have been dead by now. He re-diagnosed her with a similar tumor but one that is much less aggressive; a "pleomorphic xanthro-astrocytoma". When Jill and I spoke over the telephone, we laughed about her out-living the prognosis of two doctors so the third had to come up with a better explanation. As my wise surgeon once said, "I have learned never to say, 'never'".

I would like to see more doctors inclined to dispense the following important healing tools to all their patients:

1) the right to challenge the odds

2) the right to fight for their life,

3) the right to hopeful optimism.

Give your patients a medical hug in the form of encouragement or applauding their courage. If nothing else, give your patients permission to exceed your expectations; they just may surprise you as well as themselves.

To those of us on the receiving end of medicine, I would like more patients to give themselves the following healing tools:

1) stop considering yourselves patients,

2) start considering yourselves survivors,

3) exercise your God-given right to challenge the odds; to fight for your life; to be a hopeful optimist,

4) then, aim for the moon; you just might reach the stars.

Shortly after surgery, I stopped calling myself a patient. As you recall, I am much too impatient to bear the title. After surviving a craniotomy, I was adamant about being referred to as a survivor. Regardless of the duration of my survival, it was mine to claim.

Patient conjures up a picture of passive weakness, frailty, lack of will. The archaic meaning of "patient" is one who suffers. That definition would make the entire world patients. On the other hand, survivor implies a victory. Literally translated from the original Latin, supervivere, super meaning "over" and vivere meaning "to live", it means to "over live", or survive beyond expectations. By that definition, there are a great many survivors who are not getting their due credit.

Anyone who lives with a brain tumor is a survivor. If you are alive, you are a survivor. Allow yourself that credit even if your doctors do not say it. Do not be a patient waiting patiently for your doctors' expectations to come true. Set your own expectations and put your energies into living up to them with the best you have to give. No matter what the outcome, you will have lived - *truly lived* - without regret.

Reality is Expensive and Exhausting
The year of 1994

The reality of any illness, but especially that of a brain tumor, is not clearly defined during the crisis stage. The implications are put aside while your entire focus is concentrated on the task at hand - pure survival.

In fact, due to the nature of most brain tumors, whether a high grade glioblastoma, a low grade astrocytoma, or some of the other various tumor types, whether benign or malignant, there is an inherent characteristic about a brain tumor that makes it different from every other disease.

A brain tumor essentially attacks your very essence. It infringes upon the space the human body has reserved for personality, traits, qualities, capabilities, capacity to think, feel, reason. It touches who you are, where you reside within the physical body. Without a working brain what are we? A healthy body, a strong heart and a hearty constitution are no substitute for cognitive capacity.

If I cannot think, I cannot function. If I cannot comprehend, how can I love, know love, feel loved? I can lose my sight but still see - in my mind's eye. I can lose my hearing - and yet still hear and feel the life surrounding me. I may lose a breast or a limb and still thrive without the appendage as long as I have my mind. Without the brain's ability to function, however, meaningful life comes to an ultimate conclusion.

This ultimatum is the expensive reality of a brain tumor. It is the reality that makes brain cancer far deadlier and more devastating than many other cancers. It is what makes it *UNACCEPTABLE*.

The 1990's were declared the 'Decade of the Brain' by Ronald Reagan, then President of the United States. It was the last frontier, so to speak, in medical technology and research. Nearing the end of ten years of this proclaimed decade dedicated to research and development of brain technology, it still remains a formidable mystery, shrouded in misunderstood fear and complexity. That is unacceptable.

Reality is that this disease kills PEOPLE - mothers, fathers, sons, daughters. It leaves orphans and widows in its wake. And the harsh reality is there is little known about its cause, its cure, its prevention or management.

The reality is the statistics are just that; numbers accumulated, interpolated, extrapolated, graphed and charted to arrive at some obscure conclusion. I believe they too often become a self-fulfilling prophecy. If that is the reality, it is up to us to change it. If you understand that one table lumps ages 21 to 64 into one statistic, well that's a lot of leeway for variations (43 years leeway).

Why limit yourself or your life span with anything so nebulous?

For several years I have been trying to unite the efforts of my brain tumor world, the Central Brain Tumor Registry of the United States and the New Jersey Cancer Registry. I wanted to know how anyone could maintain meaningful statistics when so few states were actually keeping track of them or reporting them.

Just to test my theory, I called the hospital where I was diagnosed to see if I was registered and no one could find me in the system. I called the New Jersey Cancer Registry and found that brain cancer is not considered one of the top ten cancers and therefore it is not included in the published Annual Report. However, it may be requested separately. I made contact with the one statistician who indicated in 1993 the State of New Jersey was backlogged to 1988.

My immediate question to myself was - would I hang my hat, or in this case, my head, on out-of-date stats? Because it is written, is it true? Or does it become true because it has been written? The reality has been expensive for far too many.

I am grateful to the people who are working diligently to get the state of New Jersey up-to-date with accurate numbers. In 1995, the Central Brain Tumor Registry of the United States published its First Annual Report, with 12 states fully participating. All 50 states should be working as diligently to get on-line with the Registry to provide accurate data, to recognize the survival patterns and incidence, to establish awareness of the disease, ultimately, for the prevention of brain tumors.

One piece of data provided by the Central Brain Tumor Registry of the United States (CBTRUS) struck me personally. The highest incidence of brain tumors was located in four states that I had frequented throughout my life; New Hampshire where I was born and raised, Massachusetts where I spent time with friends on vacations, New Jersey where I currently live, and Rhode Island where I have gone every summer with my family.

In addition, the four counties in New Jersey where I spent the most time have the highest incidence of brain tumors. Unfortunately, the statistics didn't indicate anywhere I could go that would make me much safer.

It was only three years into the decade, 1993, when this reality came home to roost in my 'neck of the woods'. It shook the foundation of my life and ruptured my peaceful world, creating the greatest tempest I have yet to endure. To put it more bluntly, it scared the living daylights out of me. The very fact that I had made it to 1994, three months post-surgery, was incredible.

Out of every adversity comes some redeeming goodness - and mine came in many forms and from many loved ones. One of the sweetest gifts came from my Dad in a letter he sent to me shortly after my surgery. The following excerpts contain a message only a loving parent could write and one I will cherish forever:

March, 1994

My dearest daughter, Rebecca,

How many times in my mind I have written this letter to you. Finally, I will put my thoughts on paper.

This letter is to "thank" you and Warren and Krystal, and more importantly, to assure you that Mom and I love you very much. Not a day goes by without you in our thoughts and prayers, along with Warren and Krystal. Your discomfort, your anxiety, your effects from medicine, are "ours" as well and we both would "swap" in a minute your problems. Since that is beyond our control, please remember we are always available for you, Warren and Krystal and draw on us for strength twenty-four hours a day!

We are so proud of you for your courage and attitude but you have a team by your side to extend a helping hand; most important of all, Jehovah, and then the love that extends through Warren, your great loving husband, then through your daughter, your family, your friends, and your doctors.

Keep strong, keep determined because I need your strength, your keeping track of me, like you have done for so many years. Yes, I have been proud of you ever since you were born. You have brought Mom and me so many pleasant memories that no one can ever take away from us and they will last an eternity!

Now back to the 'thank you's. First, the latest card you sent Mom and me brought tears to our eyes. Your expressions of endearment have always been so 'special' to us. Every card you ever sent has been special. You have a way with words, but more important, a way of extending your love and encouragement, not only to us but so many others as well.

I keep the letter you wrote to us on our 40th anniversary on my visor in my car and so many times when I'm feeling down, I re-read your thoughts and its as if you're with me at that very moment. So thank you for all your cards, too many to mention. Thank you also for the bathrobe. During these cold zero days we've had, how this was appreciated. I use it every day.

Then there are the dinners! How many times my son-in-law, Warren, has taken us out! Thanks Warren for your generosity and hospitality. It is not taken for granted. Rebecca, keep telling your husband how fortunate you are to have his love, support and "hand" to hold. I certainly am grateful to him for being so loving and strong for you and Krystal and also for his many, many calls of encouragement and communication he has given to us. We are proud to say, he is our son and can easily say "we love him."

Thanks for being my supplier of "after shave". So many have complimented me on my "Polo" and "Photo" scents and it is all because of you and Krystal. Thanks too for both your support and concern during my heart attack. Although you are three hundred miles away, it has been so comforting to hear your concerns, it is like you are here in Manchester checking daily on your Mom and Dad.

Rebecca - So many times in my mind I have re-lived your life with us. My minds flashes back to the "joys" I had with you on Pine Street. Holding you at six weeks old. The many times Mom and I would wake up and you would be standing by our bed with a big smile. How did you get out of that crib?! Finally, I watched as you put your head down on the mattress, worked your feet up the crib walls until they reached the top, then pushed yourself up, feet first over the top crib bar, then the rest of the body 'til finally you climbed down!

I remember the many days I would come home from work at the A & P, look up to the third floor window to see your smiling face and run up three flights of stairs to be greeted by the "two-year-old doll" who had her coat and hat ready to go for a ride in Daddy's car. Yes, I remember too how you loved my home-made Italian spaghetti so much you put the sauce all over your face and head! Later I recall your school days, leading Cindy and Brian and later Jodi up the same path.

I remember when you first learned to swim. How proud we were! Then you learned to water-ski with one ski. How you attacked the water. No fears. Same way with snow skiing. Straight down the hill, no matter how steep! I often re-live the time at Massabesic Lake when you hit your head on the ice! I can still hear the crack. I think the whole lake cracked. You didn't even cry!

I remember when I hit your leg with something that shot out from the lawn mower and I had to rush you to the hospital for stitches. I was so embarrassed for my carelessness, yet I can hear you so clearly say on the surgeon's table - "It's OK Daddy, I love you so much." You have always been so strong during your adversities.

Yes, when we thought you only had a tummy ache and found out later you had appendicitis. No complaints at home or at the hospital for 15 days. How proud we were of you. How frightened we were but we got through it together.

Later when you found Warren and got married, yes, I had concerns, but I was happy that you found someone who would love you and take care of you and Warren has done that. We welcome him as our son.

Then came Krystal! What a joy! How I fell in love with my Krystal! Those eyes, that smile. Never will I forget that chubby little face that spotted Mom and me at the airport and immediately smiled or the room she willingly called "Grampy's Bedroom", the way she says the right things at the right time and takes after her mother, encouraging, and giving loving words of endearment to those close to her. How precious to us, but a jewel to you and Warren...

The letter goes on but there are no adequate words left after receiving a letter so dear to my heart, except Thank You, Dad.

Sometime later that year, I received another memorable moment from my brother, Brian. Brian and I were very close growing up. We shared a newspaper route from the time I was ten years old. We were tennis partners, skiing enthusiasts, even square-dancing buddies but most of all, best of friends.

Brian came back from a recent trip to Japan with a gift, an elegant string of pearls that he coerced a Japanese businessman to help him purchase for me, his sister. The gift was exceedingly generous and the pearls were of the highest quality but even their beauty could not match the thought and love attached to this gift. It is knowing that we are still the best of friends that I will always remember and cherish.

No matter what the cost of the reality of my new life situation, it has been worth the pain. I am living life to the fullest. I have replaced negatives with positives, fear with anticipation, anger with peace, hatred with love. I like myself, yes, very much so.

Cautious Optimism
The year of 1995

Eager to encourage my progress, Warren surprised me with a huge celebration brunch at a local restaurant in March of 1995. Not only had I reached a milestone in life, making it to forty years of age, but I had completed my chemotherapy and remained tumor-free. That was better sounding than fat-free, sugar-free, cholesterol-free and certainly sufficient reason for a celebration. With family in from the North and friends from all over the state, it was a pleasant surprise. It validated the love and support I have received from all these special friends.

In addition to my 40th milestone and the completion of all my treatments, in May we celebrated our tenth anniversary. I had a surprise of my own for Warren. I had arranged a trip to the island of Bermuda for the long over-due honeymoon we never had. Our ten years together were the happiest years of my life and in May I was feeling well enough to travel again.

Keeping with my propensity to fall under Murphy's Law: 'whatever could go wrong will', it rained for 9 out of 10 days. Not mild tropical rain, torrential down-pour rain.

We sat in the dining room on our first morning enjoying the delicious tropical fruits and breakfast buffet while sheets of water poured down the windows. Not being able to go out the first day was disappointing. By day five, we were on each other's nerves and the gray clouds were invading my spirit. I was indeed very cranky. I spent a lot of money to enjoy a special time with my husband and we found ourselves watching television cartoons in our hotel room.

Warren gets annoyed whenever I get cranky and honeymooning was becoming the farthest thing from our minds. It was more like waiting for a volcanic eruption. He had been struggling to stay positive for me. I had been fighting so hard to stay positive for him. We both had been suppressing feelings so as not to hurt the other - it finally all came pouring out. It was only after we were able to communicate our true frustrations and understand each other's feelings that we were able to get on with healing them and having a nice vacation. Not great but pleasantly nice.

We rarely fight although we often disagree. The stress of this disease places tremendous pressures on a couple's relationship and ours was no exception. The stress not only devastates your life, it can destroy your relationship with your most loved family members, your spouse, your children - if you are not careful. Be aware and be forgiving of each other. Recognize each of you are in pain and every person demonstrates pain, stress, anxiety in different ways.

One day it was raining but only lightly, so we began to walk the beaches from Elbow Beach all the way down to

Horseshoe Bay. We talked out our feelings and cleared the air of our fears and frustrations, as well as the rain. Warren did not want to risk going out on a Moped with me and given the fact that I already had one Moped accident in Bermuda, I was inclined to agree. So we were forced to see the island through the windows of the Bermuda bus system, not exactly romantic, but it was efficient. While I had been to Bermuda many times and knew my way around, I was disappointed for Warren. He could not see the beauty and enjoy the tiny island the way I had hoped because the rain cast a gloomy grayness over the whole island. There was a gray cloud cover for all but one day - our last. He did not get to swim in the beautiful blue azure ocean, see the parrot fish up close in the water, he did not get to take in the breath-taking views, the panoramic view from Gibbs lighthouse.

He was terrific in his attitude of "let's just make the best of it." I was the one pouting and complaining and making him miserable, but Warren doesn't let me get away with that for long and soon I shook off my disappointment and we enjoyed our time together. After all, that is why we came here, to spend quality time together.

My friend, Janet, had recommended a place for our anniversary dinner. I had never been to The Courtyard restaurant that was part of the Bermuda Culinary Institute. It was a dining experience we will both cherish and the evening brought us back to the love that has kept us together for over ten years. We sat in the open courtyard with hibiscus and frangipani, fragrant, tropical floral trees creating a private dining room outdoors. The staff are students at the Culinary Institute and attend to your every need, preparing many exotic dishes at your table. The food was magnificent, the ambiance impeccable, and although clouds loomed overhead, we were not rained on during our romantic evening.

Having been to Bermuda many times before, I had many fond memories and friends living there whom I had not seen in over twenty years. One of the fondest memories from our trip was meeting up with Randy and Edie Wells, my friends from Devonshire, Bermuda. Over twenty years earlier, they had opened their home and their hearts to me and they have remained in my heart ever since. After talking to Randy on the telephone, we made reservations at the Waterlot Inn for dinner: a charming restaurant on the Bermuda waterfront; a place with special memories from long ago.

I was afraid for my friends to see me after the trauma of my brain tumor treatments, loss of hair and excess weight, thinking, what if they don't recognize me, what if we have nothing to talk about? On the other hand, I did not know when or if I would see them again and I so wanted to see them - it was worth any embarrassment I felt. Upon spotting each other, we recognized each other immediately and I was welcomed with all the warmth and sunshine I had been deprived of during my stay on the island. It truly is the people of Bermuda that make this tiny island so special to me.

Warren and Randy met for the first time and soon were engrossed in conversation as if they knew each other for a lifetime. Edie and I compared notes on our kids and looked at photos and talked effortlessly. It was as if we picked up where we left off twenty years ago. I don't know when, but I do know I WILL go back and I am sure the sun will shine for us next time.

Throughout 1995, we proceeded with a cautious optimism as every three month scan showed no tumor, no sign of recurrence. It is an odd feeling to be afraid to be too elated each time the scan results are good. It is hard to not be able to do more than breathe a sigh of relief. But life continues on one day at a time and soon a week has passed, a month has slipped away, and before you know it, another year is on the horizon. More positive action was on my horizon.

It was at my final chemotherapy session, that I spotted a poster taped up on the wall advertising an organization called Chemo Care. Chemo Care is an independent organization dedicated to helping people dealing with chemotherapy. I called immediately and was told they would contact a brain tumor survivor who would call me on the telephone. In a day or two I received a call from a young woman who had survived a brain tumor similar to mine.

Dawn was young and effervescent and a survivor of an Anaplastic Astrocytoma. She glowed with good health and a bubbling energy. Under the terms of the organization, we were allowed to speak three times - but it only took one minute with Dawn to feel better. She was so full of life and a confident attitude, a positively determined spirit.

Chemo Care also sent me a brochure which would improve my survival efforts immensely. It was a flyer from the Central New Jersey Brain Tumor Support Group which led me to another path leading me to many remarkable people and incredible life experiences. I eagerly, but cautiously, entered the conference room donated by the church for the support meetings. There were three people seated and already in discussion when I entered alone. I was offered a seat by a gentleman named, Stan. Patricia Phillips, a neurosurgical nurse affiliated with a local hospital was leading the group in discussion. At my first meeting I soon learned I was the only brain tumor survivor present. A quorum of one, does not a group make, I thought silently to myself, but these people were so warm and welcoming I instantly felt I had found friends.

I returned the following month. The group meets on the first Thursday of each month and soon I met other brain tumor survivors. It was so encouraging to have a place to talk with people who actually knew what I was talking about or what I was feeling. It was great to have a facilitator like Patty who, as a neurosurgical nurse, knew the other side of the medical issues. She had been running the group meetings for two years when I joined. Stan told me that his wife, Virginia, would eventually be re-joining our little group again. She had taken some time off after they lost their dear son, Matthew, to a brain tumor.

A few months later, I met Virginia for the first time and felt I had met a soul mate, a friend forever. We seemed to connect in the way we thought about things and we had the same driving passion to do something positive about this horrible disease. Working with Patty, we began planning meetings with specialty speakers who would talk to the group and allow for questions and answers.

We feverishly put together new flyers with the most eye-catching colors; lime-green, fuchsia, magenta, canary yellow - in hopes that more people would notice them. Stan had set up a data base on his home computer and we began doing monthly mailings to members.

A graphic artist friend designed a poster which we distributed to hospitals and doctors' offices notifying others of the free services offered through the Central New Jersey Brain Tumor Support Group. People began coming from New Jersey, New York, Pennsylvania. Doctors and other medical professionals offered their services, free of charge, as our meetings are free to all who wish to attend. This is a service which not only benefits patients but the medical community as well.

The group gradually began to grow - not just in numbers but in dynamics. We began to evolve from an ad hoc support group to an organization determined to make a difference. We drew speakers who willingly donated their time and expertise to assist our members. We had an herbalist talk about alternative medicine, a yoga specialist demonstrate (with group participation) yoga exercises, a pharmacist talk about brain tumor medications, a bio-technical PhD who does brain tumor research present a slide overview of latest research and technology as well as a preview of future treatments. Our group became keenly aware of the need for funding not only to continue its own efforts, but to ultimately fund research for a cure.

Through the local hospital, resources were provided to host a local conference for brain tumors survivors.

Doctors, surgeons, radiologists and oncologists participated in a full day's program along with a luncheon for the over 500 in attendance.

In addition, the group provides support for entire families dealing with the trauma of a brain tumor, has break-out meetings for care-givers and children, and schedules end of the year celebration activities. We developed a Resource Center of books, periodicals, and resource materials available for brain tumors survivors. In 1994 we created a ribbon representing our dedication to the brain tumor cause. We wanted a symbol that indicated our commitment to finding a cure for brain tumors. The significance of the ribbon was explained as follows:

The Story of the Ribbon

> *Having a brain tumor is like living with a cloud over your head. With dedication and research, we know that within the cloud we will find a silver lining that will eradicate brain tumors forever.*
>
> *A gold star on a silver ribbon identifies a brain tumor survivor. A silver star identifies the wearer as a family member, friend, or supporter.*

The ribbons have been requested and distributed to brain tumor survivors and their supporters throughout the United States, Canada, and many places abroad.

My neuro-surgeon makes sure he wears his ribbon on his lapel every time I go to his office for my periodic scan review. I truly appreciate his effort to show his support.

In addition to the ribbons, we organized the Support Group into a full fledged organization with non-profit status.

We were graciously provided pro bono legal and accounting services by two generous members of the community who want to support our efforts. Virginia is an incredible lady with lots of great ideas and talents and a most compassionate nature. Everyone gravitates to her because of her caring personality and she has been extremely instrumental in winning the services of these professionals. Because of our incorporated status we were able to do a fund-raiser to raise funds towards the on-going function of the group as well as moving towards our objective to provide funds for research.

We had tee-shirts made up with BIG BOLD BLACK letters that say, of course, **THAT'S UNACCEPTABLE** - with a bright yellow sun above it to imply hope and healing. My surgeon has promised to wear his shirt to the top of Mount Ranier in Washington State and dedicate the climb to all brain tumor patients. I have been promised a picture to commemorate the event.

The group has been a truly beneficial experience in dealing with a brain tumor. We have provided services to over 500 brain tumor survivors, their families and friends, as well as the medical profession. Doctors and hospitals refer their patients and those who accept our invitation to join us at one of our meetings are usually uplifted and inspired to do better. I am personally proud of the group and all the professionals who have gratuitously supported it.

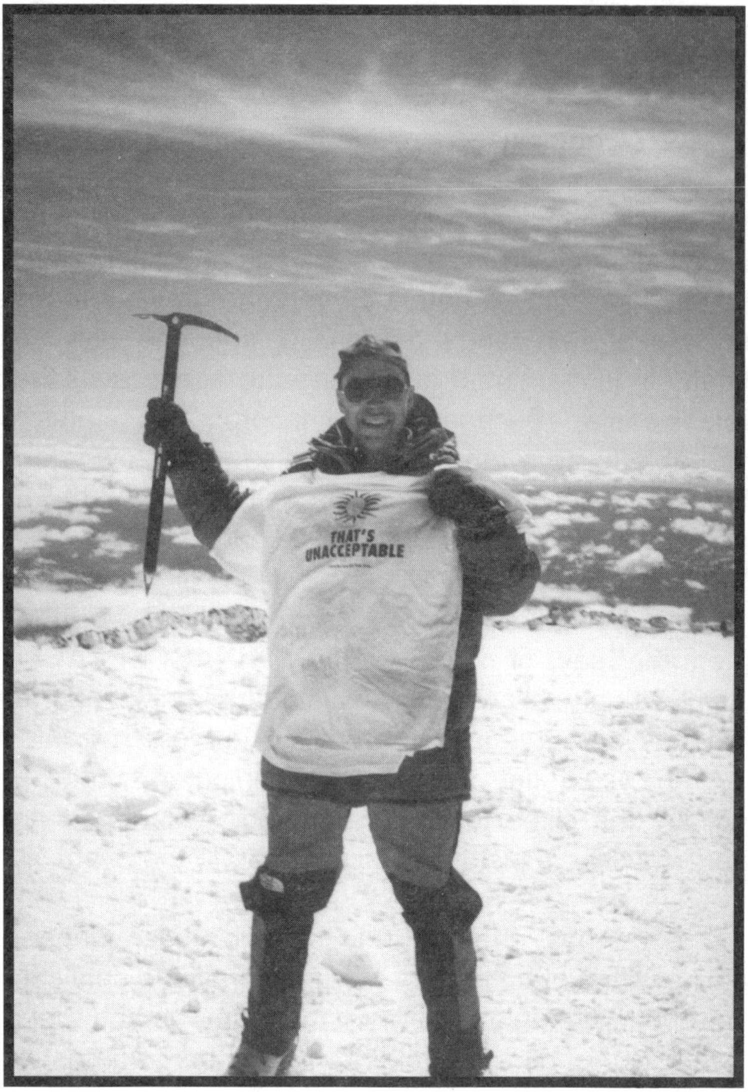

Dr. Beyerl - Columbia Crest - Mt. Ranier

On July 2, 1997 Dr. Beyerl reached the summit of Mt. Ranier at an altitude of 14,410 feet. He dedicated his climb to all brain tumor patients. With doctors like this, we can all reach greater heights!

During Brain Tumor Awareness Week, the group nominated me as their Survivor of the Year and asked me to share my story of survival. I am happy to say we now have many long term survivors of many types of brain tumors. While it is always sad to lose some of our members to this disease, we have a place to share even our grief and frustrations. It is a place where you are welcomed warmly and understood. The problems are discussed but the focus is on solutions. It has been proven that those who attend support groups generally do better in their recovery. Our group is a fine example of improving the quantity and quality of life for those dealing with a brain tumor.

In addition to the local support group meetings, I was introduced to the Internet which provides access to a Brain Tumor List. This list includes over 1,000 participants who can exchange information, support, current treatment and protocol, questions, answers, hopes, fears, frustrations. It is open, honest, brutally honest at times, but professional and overall positive. It is a place to find answers from all over the globe. One morning I signed on to get a message from a doctor in Australia who read one of my postings. He was so happy to see my name, as he had evaluated me during his internship in Boston, Massachusetts at Massachusetts General Hospital. He had later received a grant to return to Australia and open a brain tumor clinic. It was exciting to be remembered by him and to learn of his activities to help others.

I have met many special people over the Internet and recently many of us met face-to-face at a conference in New York City. The conference was sponsored by the

Brain Tumor Society located in Boston, Massachusetts. The conference was to assist brain tumor survivors and their families and friends with information provided by the top professionals in the field from all over the entire country. The work done by the Brain Tumor Society in the fight against brain tumors is truly inspirational.

They have provided funding for many worthy research grants as the one above. The organization truly inspires "Hope for a Cure" and channels their efforts to that end. Bonnie Feldman, its founder and driving force, works endlessly to make a difference and I have great admiration for her success. She truly has made a tremendous impact upon brain tumor survivors and the medical society in which we find ourselves. Without the work of people like Bonnie, Patty, and Virginia, we would still be in the dark ages in the fight against brain tumors. It has been a privilege to play a small part in this effort.

Through the Central NJ Brain Tumor support group I was introduced to Suzanne Levy who has worked with a local chapter of the American Cancer Society. Each May, they hold a fund raiser to benefit the American Cancer Society. It was a special treat to be invited to be a model in the Celebration of Life Fashion show as the first brain tumor survivor to participate in this annual event. We were given a make-over with hair and make-up done by professionals and designer evening wear from Saks Fifth Avenue.

My escort was a charming young man who had survived cancer. It was a fabulous surprise to find out we had worked together for years by telephone and were now meeting for the first time at this gala event. At the conclusion of the show, the Cancer Society asked me to include my daughter, Krystal, on the final walk down the runway. She was delighted and Warren was proud of both of us. What a celebration to our new life!

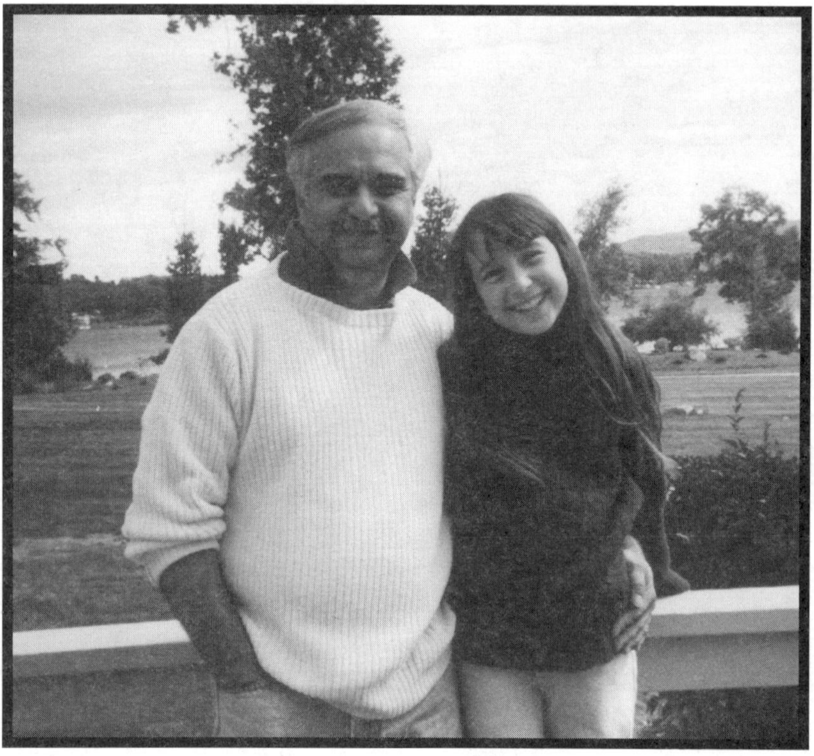

Warren and Krystal
At Lake Winnepasaukee, New Hampshire

Resolving the Unresolvable
The Year of 1996

The year of 1996 arrived with great promise. It was a full year since I had taken any formal medical treatment. I was improving slowly but surely every day. Knowing I wanted and needed a connection to my family and my home in New England, Warren offered to buy me a condominium on Lake Winnepasaukee. We had spent many summer vacations at the lake and found a lovely place we decided to buy. The contract went through, the financing was approved, the interest rate was set, and our plan to close on the deal was long in coming but finally scheduled. One week before the closing date we were handed some information which killed the deal. It was heart-breaking to have come so close to a dream only to have it shattered. I had spent months taking care of all the details and felt wiped out both physically and emotionally. In hind sight I can call it a blessing in disguise but when it was occurring, it felt like being kicked when you are already down.

This became my year to resolve matters which had previously been unresolvable. After my surgery I was still allowed to drive. Warren, however, was concerned about my having to use a gear shift so he gave my car to his niece and bought me a new Acura with automatic everything. We had it for about three months. Warren was leaving the house to play an early game of tennis when he found two 'guys' trying to break into my car. He ran after them as they fled to get away and caught one by the foot when he fell. They jumped in the get-away car and sped off to whatever dark places these kind of people reside. Two days later they returned and vandalized the car by breaking all the locks and door handles. The police said it was an act of retaliation. It took months to get it fixed.

In 1996, I awoke from what I thought was a major bad dream. It was unusual for me to dream at all since phenobarbital inhibits the REM stage of sleep. But, the dream was so real, I thought someone was stealing my car. At 5:00 a.m. I jumped out of bed, another unusual occurrence, and ran to the window. No car. I ran to the back window. No car. I grabbed my robe and slippers and rushed down the stairs telling myself it was only a dream. I opened the door and walked up and down the driveway, then out to the street. No car.

There I stood looking up to the heavens in the middle of the street in the middle of the wee morning hours in my nightgown and robe saying, "What else can they do to me?" "When is enough, enough?" The answer was yet to come. After a week my car was recovered. It was smashed and all my belongings were stolen. My property had been violated. After two months, dealing with our local auto-body shop who was the only one profiting from this car, the Acura was fixed and nearly new again.

After its return, I bought the "club" and parked up near the garage under the motion detector lights. Warren would park his car behind mine. A few weeks later an attempt to get into the car for the fourth time occurred. It made no sense and now not only was my car in danger, but my privacy had been invaded. These guys would come all the way into my yard with no way of getting the car out, just to destroy it. I called the detectives and insisted they take fingerprints that were left on the window of the vehicle. I asked for extra street patrol to ensure the safety of the neighborhood. Nothing turned up in the fingerprint files but I have not had any further problems. After all the police reports, auto-body visits, insurance claim forms, it was about time this was finally resolved.

In addition to my car being stolen and vandalized, 1996 brought with it a few more aggravations that required resolution. Krystal's fourth grade teacher was causing tremendous stress and pressure on our entire family. She was insistent that Krystal was intentionally not paying attention. She refused to recognize the impact my illness had on Krystal's ability to focus and function. She used intimidation, humiliation, and degradation. She isolated Krystal and encouraged negative peer pressure. Warren and I repeatedly tried to reason with her to no avail.

We went to the principal with little resolution. We went to Pupil Services with no satisfaction. I finally went to the Superintendent of the school district. Still, the abuse continued. This teacher had tenure and apparently little was going to be done.

We were forced to the wall. I was tired and out of ammunition to fight the system. So I documented everything. I wrote the dates, the comments, the actions. I interviewed children in the class and wrote statements confirming the information. I put it all in a detailed letter and addressed it to the Principal and copied the Director of Pupil Services as well as the Superintendent. I concluded my documentation with the simple fact that if this treatment did not cease immediately, our attorney would be advised to take action. We concluded the school year without further incident. The matter was resolved but the damage had already been done. It would take the rest of 1996 to re-build Krystal's self-esteem. It would take a new teacher with new insight to remedy the injustice. With time, this too was resolved.

Krystal is now stronger, self-confidant, and shining in her work. She learned a life lesson - life is not fair, it is not just, it just is - and we must learn to deal with it. Some people are not nice. We do not have to accept it and we don't have to like it but we do have to deal with it.

After this ordeal Krystal asked for a kitten. Knowing how much she had suffered through the recent months and how hard she had tried, I convinced Warren to at least let her put a proposal together for him to consider. Being an engineer, he was impressed with the 10-page proposal she presented to him. Against his own reservations he agreed to allow her a kitten.

Since I was severely allergic to cats all my life, my herbalist recommended a homeopathic liquid for animal dander. We also got a special product to wash the cat monthly. In all honesty, I believe that it is impossible to be allergic to anyone you love and I love that cat. I have not had a serious allergic reaction since little Demi arrived in our home.

This little rascal has added more laughter and love to our home and healed an aching heart in Krystal and her mother. Murphy and Demi adore each other and kiss and lick each other's face every morning. They play tag running through my dining room and living room but the joy they give us is worth it.

In three years we had not taken Krystal out on a school night because of all the demands of homework and keeping up. We felt it was time to do something fun together as a family. We got tickets to see Victor Borga, the pianist/comedian who was doing a show at the New Jersey State Theater. We laughed and enjoyed Krystal's laughter. It was the laughter of a child - the pure delight of a giggling child. We took her to dinner and thoroughly enjoyed the evening. It is Krystal's dream to be a comedienne someday and it is her mother's hope that she will continue to play piano. This show was a hopeful inspiration for combining the two talents. Move over Victor, your successor is coming!

When we returned home we found the basement sitting under four inches of water. The dog and cat stared in wide-eyed amazement with a look on both of their faces that said, "We didn't do it, honest, we didn't." It was just another little issue to be resolved in 1996. Sometimes you just get the feeling you're never gonna get a break. But life has a way of compensating for all the mishaps and the little trials. After dealing with a brain tumor, in the grand scheme of things, what does it matter?

In September of 1996 I celebrated my third anniversary from surgery and diagnosis of a brain tumor. The National Brain Tumor Foundation interviewed me for a Survival Story to be included in their Summer Issue of SEARCH - their newsletter. It is a beautiful, hopeful article which has generated more responses than I could have imagined. People wrote and called and e-mailed me from all over the country and parts of Canada. It has been my reward to share my hope and optimism with others.

With the gracious permission of the National Brain Tumor Foundation, this story of survival "Recovery Unlimited" is reprinted to be shared with all. For more information on the National Brain Tumor Foundation call toll-free 1-800-934-CURE.

Survivor's Story
Rebecca Libutti: Recovery Unlimited

In 1993, when doctors told Rebecca Libutti that the type of brain tumor she had could end her life in a year, she blurted out the first words that came to her mind: "That's Unacceptable!"

Today, three years later, her words are emblazoned on a t-shirt which her neurosurgeon wears as a tribute to Rebecca's indomitable spirit.

"When I was given my prognosis," Rebecca recalls, "I said it was unacceptable and that's been my attitude all along."

At the time of her diagnosis, Rebecca was 38, enjoying her life as a wife and mother as well as her full time career as manager for a large insurance firm in New Jersey. The brain tumor - a glioblastoma multiforme grade 4 - arrived in her life unannounced and unwelcome.

"The only warning I had," she says, "was when I woke up on a Monday morning ready to go to work and I had the most incredible headache of my life. I couldn't lift my head off the pillow."

After three days of initially being treated for a sinus infection, Rebecca had a CT (computerized tomography) scan which revealed a mass on her brain. She was immediately sent to Overlook Hospital to meet with a physician. "They told me there was a room and a neurosurgeon waiting for me at the hospital," Rebecca says. "That was the first and last time I've had a doctor waiting for me."

When she recovered from surgery, Rebecca went through 35 standard radiation treatments and took a combination of chemotherapeutic drugs including BCNU, procarbazine (PCB) and vincristine.

But that's not all she did.

"From the very beginning," Rebecca says, "I determined that I would do everything I could do medically to help myself, but I was not going to just stop there. I would do everything else I could find to promote the healing process and what I call the recovering process."

Consequently, she searched out other brain tumor survivors for support, investigated and used herbal alternatives, began massage therapy -- and walked her dog, a 95-pound Labrador retriever named Murphy Brown. "One of my philosophies was that if I kept moving the brain tumor couldn't get me," Rebecca says laughing. "So within a month after my surgery I was walking my dog two miles a day."

While she takes full charge of her recovery today, Rebecca admits that it can be initially difficult for brain tumor survivors to direct their own care. "In the beginning," she says, "you do what you're advised to do because you can't even pronounce the name of what you've got."

"When I started out," she continues, "all I had was a scrap of paper with the name of my tumor written on it and I went from there. I started doing research and read over 75 books in the first year after my surgery. I searched all over the country talking to every well-known doctor I could find and I didn't just get second opinions, I got third opinions too. God granted me the gift of time, and I was going to use it in saving my life."

Eventually, Rebecca signed on to the Internet and used it to share information with other brain tumor survivors. She also asked questions of participating physicians, one of whom directed her to a medical text (*Radiation Injury to the Nervous System*) when she was researching the effects of radiation. "I'm not a medical professional," Rebecca says, "but I do know what I have and I can decipher enough from the medical texts to put intelligent questions together. Then I can take the questions to my radiologist or my doctor and get answers about my case specifically."

As part of her investigations, Rebecca also searched out an herbal medicine practitioner to help her cope with chemotherapy. Initially, she used aloe vera juice and acidophilus/bifidophilis to calm her stomach, and liquid chlorophyll to build up her blood. "I was one of the few people in my group," Rebecca says, "who went through the harshness of the chemotherapy treatments and I never had my blood count drop below acceptable levels throughout the whole 11 months."

With her knowledge and confidence in complementary therapies growing, Rebecca began to add to her repertoire of treatments. She now follows a regimen that includes a number of herbs and multi vitamins to boost her immune system -- and she drinks two quarts of water a day.

Rebecca points out, however, that it is important to research and evaluate any complementary therapies.

"It's not just a matter of buying herbs and things in bottles," she says. "Go to a real herbal practitioner, not just someone in a health food store. My practitioner has been invaluable to me because I've learned about what I need individually. She's not only helped me in getting past the diagnosis stage but also in surviving day to day. For instance, I can now tell when I'm having an allergic reaction to mold rather than thinking it has something to do with the brain tumor."

Besides strengthening her body, Rebecca has built up her mental muscles as well. She attends the New Jersey Central Brain Tumor Support Group and she finds a great deal of strength in her family. "My husband Warren has been an absolute rock," she says. "His determination has encouraged me to never give up. I've also been blessed to have an extended family on both sides who are wonderfully supportive and I have a tremendous network of friends. All put together it becomes a very positive environment for survival."

Her daughter, Krystal, who is now 10 years old, has also inspired Rebecca's recovery. "I decided that no matter what would come ahead I would spend time doing wonderful, happy things with my daughter," Rebecca says. As a result of that decision, mother and daughter have embarked on projects such as building a doll house, planting a rose garden and making porcelain dolls. “Because of my daughter,” she adds, “I’ve also started taking piano lessons for the first time. It’s a wonderful therapy because it requires you to coordinate eyes, hands, feet and memory simultaneously to create beautiful music.”

Like other brain tumor survivors, Rebecca has learned the value -- and the challenge -- of taking life “one day at a time.”

“Everyone says to live one day at a time,” she observes, “but our world isn’t set up that way. People tell you to enjoy the moment but then they ask ‘What are you doing next week?’ So I’ve had to learn to just think about the things that make me happy and the things I have to be grateful for in each day.”

“You can’t expect every day to be wonderful,” she adds. “You can’t wake up every day smiling like some Barbie doll. But you can expect that no matter how bad you feel at the moment, that moment will pass and you’ll have a chance to have another good moment.”

This article was reprinted in its entirety with permission from the National Brain Tumor Foundation.

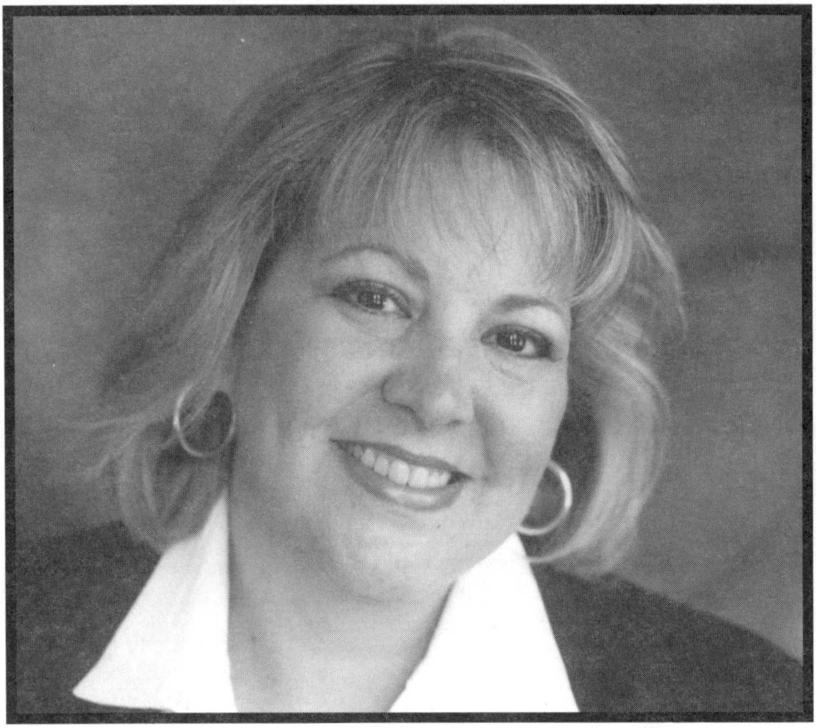

Photograph courtesy of Gene Gabelli of Gabelli Studios

Rebecca Libutti is Alive and Well
And Living With Her Family In New Jersey

Failure is Not an Option
The Year of 1997 - ad infinitum

I feel like I am sitting on top of the crest of a huge wave. It is strong, powerful. It is terrifying but exhilarating and challenging my abilities. It has pushed me and raised me up high. I feel like shouting in triumph -"I rode the wave - I conquered the fear!" But have I?

Honestly, I am not sure - no longer sure of anything. The older I get the less I know for a certainty. The wiser I become the more I know what I do not know for sure. Life and its unpredictability will continue to hold me in suspense. What I have become sure of is only what matters to me. I know I love my God, my faith. I know I love my family, each and every one of them. I know my life has been good, very good. I know failure is not an option. It is, however, a nagging possibility that helps to keep me focused on being grateful for each new day.

'"Failure," it is said, "is not falling down, it is staying down." I may fall, I may stumble, I may find myself in the depths of despair. But I will never stay there. I am determined to live each and every moment of my life to the fullest. I will never whimper out of this world. If I go, it will be kicking and fighting and laughing in the face of adversity until that moment when I can finally exhale and sleep in peace, free from this enemy for good.

Not one of us here on planet earth knows how long we have to spend here. The difference between success and failure in life is not defined by longevity, power, or wealth. Health does not determine our success. Living life to the best of our ability, helping our fellowman, living with grace and honor and dignity, true to yourself and the One who put you here, that is success. To know that when you are gone, you have left behind some imprint of your existence that has made this world a better place.

Many years ago, I wrote a book of favorite expressions and sayings. In it I summarized, "My life; a collection of sweet nothings, whispered into the ear of humanity".

Once again, Jimmy Buffet comes to my mind with the lyrics to one of his songs, "Some of its magic and some of its tragic, but I had a good life all the way."

And the journey continues . . .

False Hope?

In August, 1996, my Mother's family held their 11th family reunion at Hilton Head, South Carolina. All nine of my Mom's brothers' and sisters' families gathered together for a wonderful refreshing re-connecting of a family spread over the country from New Hampshire to Washington, and many states in-between. There were at least five generations represented in this loving and diverse Greek family with ages ranging from 24 months to 83 years. We took long bike rides together, played tennis, took a group sailing ship while others went deep sea fishing. We returned to our cluster of condominiums to meet at the pool. We had cocktail hours at each others' condominiums and attended the big family dinner at an elegant resort, complete with dancing and pictures being flashed everywhere.

One of my cousins is a medical doctor, specializing in infectious disease. While sitting at the pool one afternoon, he and I talked about my health concerns and my hopes. I took this opportunity to ask him a question I so often wanted to ask the many medical professionals I met along the way. "Why do so many doctors seem to have a hard time offering their patients hope? Is there an unwritten code that doesn't allow for hope as part of the healing process?" He explained to me that many doctors do not want to offer 'false hope'; an explanation I had heard before.

Ah, yes, false hope. I couldn't get it out of my mind. What is false about hope? How could a hopeful feeling be false or even possibly detrimental? If you gave someone hope, what is the worst that could happen? If they did better than expected, then it helped. If they did worse than expected, would they be better off without hope? I quickly found the questions but no satisfaction in the answers.

So I sat at my computer one day and wrote this poem, dedicating it to my dear cousin, Steve, along with his universal medical colleagues. I hope, truly hope, you can find it within your power to offer this valuable healing medicine and never consider it false or misleading. If I hadn't met a doctor who gave me the right to hope early in my journey, this journey of a thousand miles may have never taken me this far.

False Hope - the Oxymoron

Hope is Hope, a feeling of trust,
Against all odds, we do what we must.

Hope is a confident expectation,
Not a guarantee of a realization.

It thrives in the soul, beats in the heart
But Oh, what strength it does impart.

There is nothing false about this feeling,
It has no limit, it has no ceiling.

Hope inspires determination
To reach a dream with anticipation.

No you cannot infuse it,
You cannot draw it into a vial to use it.
You cannot measure it by rads
or take its pulse when you're tired or sad.

But drink it in with great desire
Its medicinal power can raise you higher.

Hope is truly free insurance.
It indemnifies with utmost assurance.

It rises above deep despair.
It lifts the hearts of those who care.

It is not a panacea or a cure for every ill.
It is a source of optimism, a place to find your will.

When stress and fear are set in motion,
Hope proves true as a stronger emotion.

No, you dare not deny it,
You must not defy it.
Eternal, they say it springs,
Of promises it softly sings.

It cannot be false anymore than false sorrow,
For its basic belief, is there's always tomorrow.

If hope is false then surely I guess,
There must be false hopelessness.

What would it mean to have false hopelessness?
Perhaps that indeed it was true hopefulness.

So let's turn it around or inside out,
Because hope is something we cannot live without.

Only an oxymoron would call it untrue,
Especially when hope is alive in you.

* * * * * * * * * * *

May you have Health, Happiness and Hope

Dedicated to my doctors who inspired me with hope and to those who were afraid to give me 'false hope'; may we all share in the healing power of hopeful optimism.

The Other Side
My Husband's Perspective

This portion is reserved for the time when my husband can tell his side of the story, as only a loving care-giver can do. It is a painful endeavor which, when he is ready, will flow with all the love and emotion he has reserved for helping me survive. Until then, my friends, know that you are not alone, nor forgotten.

To order additional copies of *That's Unacceptable*, fill out the coupon below and mail it with your check or money order to:

Krystal Publishing
P. O. Box 221
Martinsville, NJ 08836

Please send me _____ copies of Rebecca Libutti's book, *That's Unacceptable*, at $19.95 per copy (Canadian price is $24.95). Shipping and handling charges in the amount of $3.00 should also be included. New Jersey residents must include state sales tax of $1.20. Please allow 4 - 6 weeks for delivery.

Name ______________________________

Address ______________________________

City ______________________________

State ______________ Zip ______________

In case we have questions about your order, please include your telephone number __________________

Number of Books______ times $19.95 = __________

Shipping and Handling = 3.00

NJ Sales Tax (if applicable) = (1.20)

Total amount enclosed = __________